MW01631304

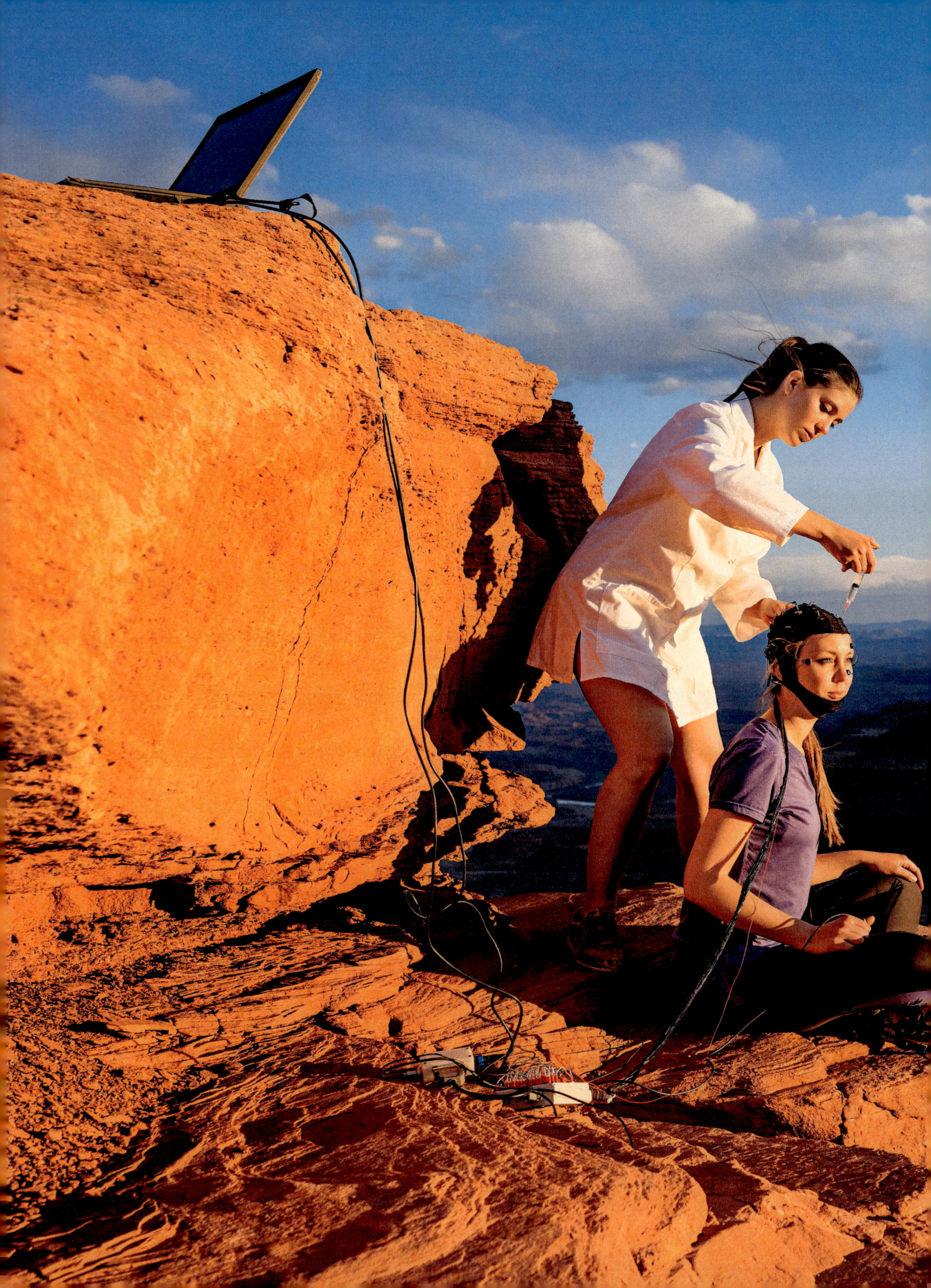

THE BRAIN
Discover the Ways Your Mind Works

Julia Sklar

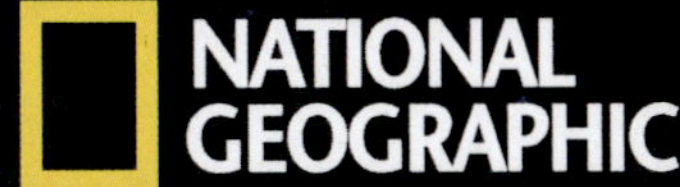

WASHINGTON, D.C.

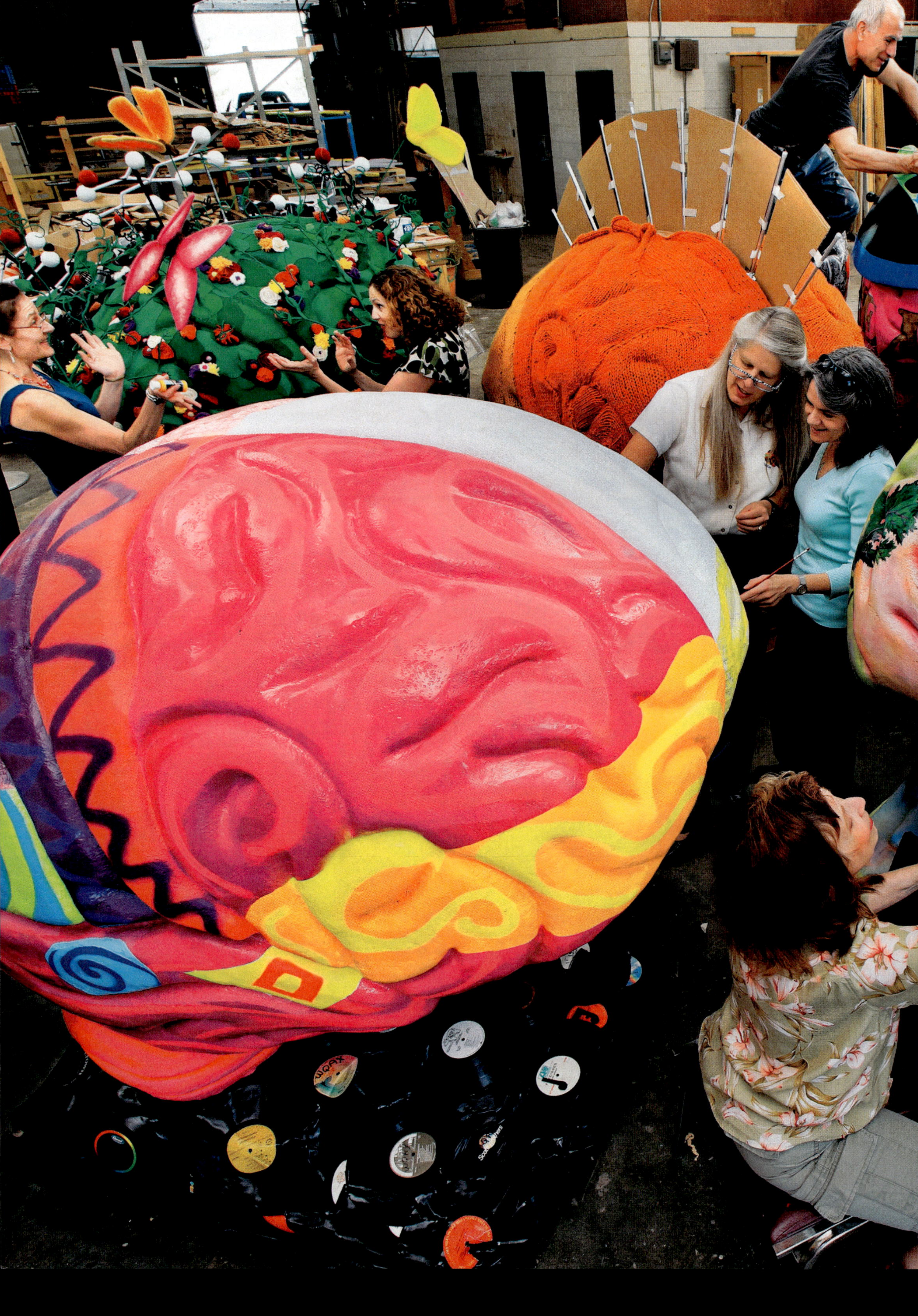

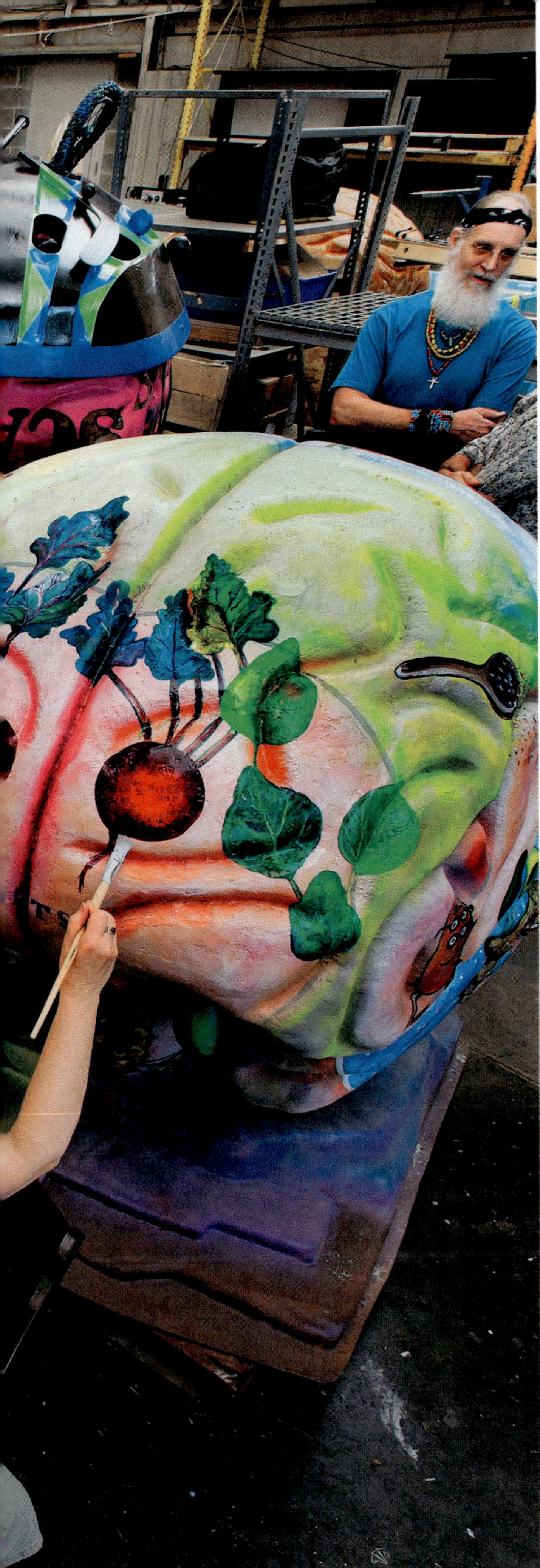

CONTENTS

Artists create anatomically correct human brain sculptures in Bloomington, Indiana, to raise awareness about brain health. *Previous Pages:* As a woman relaxes in Dead Horse Point State Park in Utah, a researcher injects conductive solution into an EEG cap to find out how brain waves differ in nature versus urban environments.

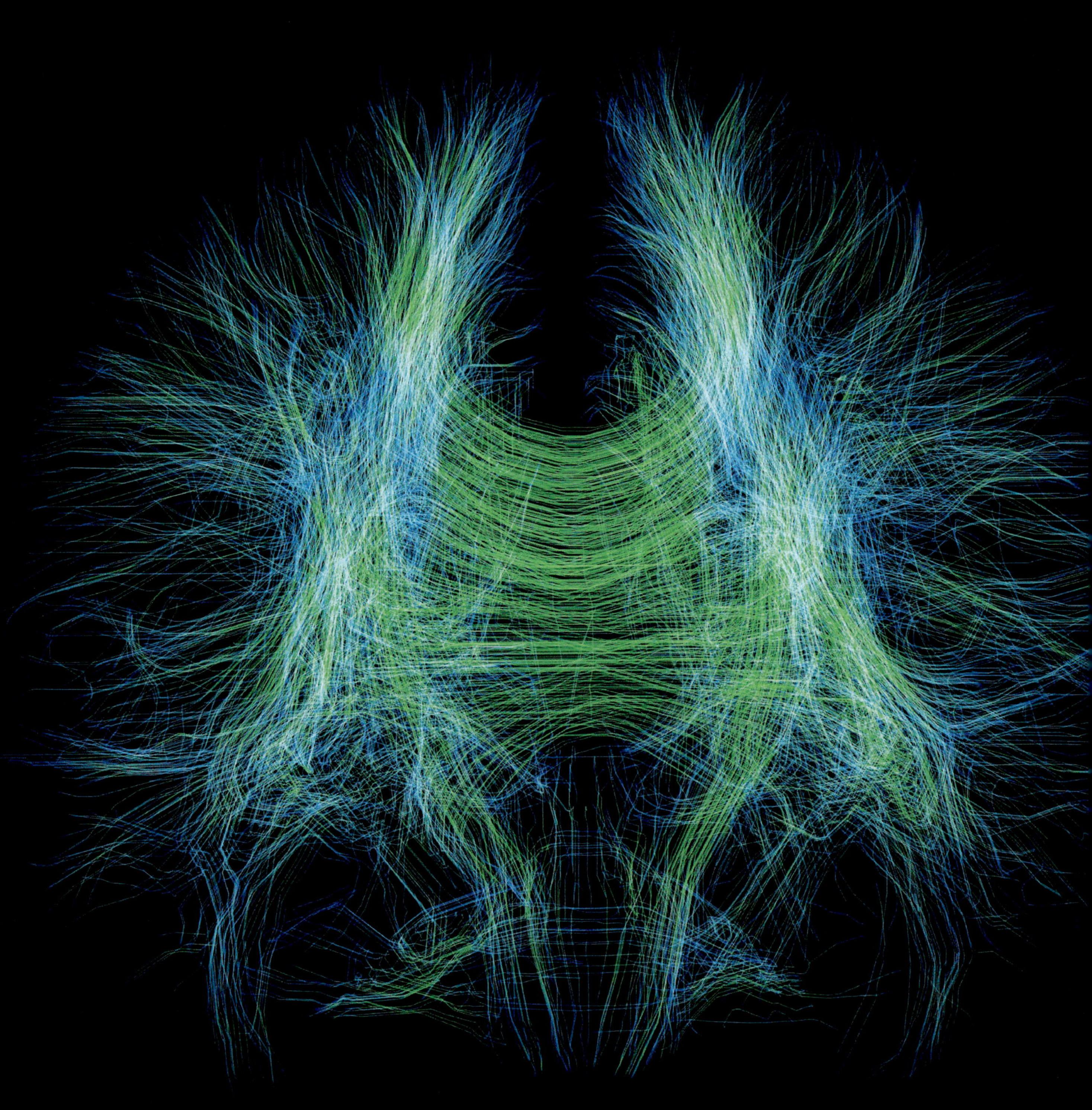

Inside the visible tissue of the brain is an organized network of ghostly nerve pathways, conveyors of information. New imaging techniques, like this diffusion tensor scan that measures the direction of water diffusion, allow scientists to see how these networks orient themselves.

INTRODUCTION

THE NEW ERA OF NEUROSCIENCE

Understanding the brain is the final frontier of human biology. This three-pound (1.4-kg) organ that presides over our bodies remains as elusive, complex, and diverse as it is universally commanding. Our discrete understanding of the brain is fairly new, as the first academic departments devoted to studying neuroscience didn't appear until the 1960s. For the next 40 years, brain science was hyper-focused on establishing the basics: What's a neuron? How do brain cells communicate with each other? What are the brain's functional areas that map onto behaviors?

That foundation supports today's researchers as they ask deeper questions: How is it possible that we perceive the world differently from each other despite having the same basic hardware? Can we manipulate our own brains? What makes us human? There is immense scientific diversity in how these questions may get answered. Studying the molecular underpinnings of the brain, for example, is almost a distinct pursuit from studying the brain as a complex computational machine in its own right. And both are different still from how neuropsychology seeks to understand behavior through brain function.

Having more, and better, exploratory tools has also led to more, and better, questions about the object being explored. Neuroscience would not be what it is today without advances in technology. In the early 2000s, functional magnetic resonance imaging (fMRI) began opening windows into the activity of the brain's regions, a huge advance over studying the static brain through a microscope. And just as the internet lets people with unique brain disorders find each other instead of living in isolation, it also helps researchers find these individuals, pushing brain science beyond case studies and into the realm of more robust, large-scale, longitudinal work.

There are no simple answers to the questions neuroscientists now pose, and that's both a great and terrifying thing. It's time to redraw the map that plots the brain as a simple organ with siloed regions for major functions—motor control, language, memory, sensation, and decision-making—because all of these areas talk to each other, and rely on dense, meshed networks to do so. With information zooming in every direction among 86 billion neurons, it's incredible that anything works at all, and yet—for the most part—it does. Welcome to the complex world of the interconnected brain.

The Interconnected Brain

If you've ever seen a diagram of the brain divided into a few sections labeled with discrete human behaviors, forget about it. The living brain, a mass of 86 billion intertwined neurons, isn't that plainly or cleanly organized. The actions, emotions, reflexes, memories, and so much more that color your life come from immense networks of brain areas working together, sometimes across blurred borders and multiple functions.

This illustration will help you keep track of the brain's dizzying interconnectedness as you read the following pages, with areas colored in hues corresponding to the chapters that reference them (some, with stripes, appear in more than one chapter).

■ CHAPTER 1

Perception, how we uniquely experience the world, relies on information "highways" in the brain. Differences here can lead to extraordinary sensations or an inability to recognize faces.

■ CHAPTER 2

Flavor seems like it comes from the mouth when we chew, but it's actually the brain pulling many simultaneous strings to create a multisensory experience.

■ CHAPTER 3

Pain is an ever present necessity for safely navigating the world, yet the complex networks that give rise to it can go awry, all while the brain itself feels no pain.

■ CHAPTER 4

Consciousness is the final frontier of neuroscience. To understand how consciousness works, start by breaking it into a set of much smaller human experiences.

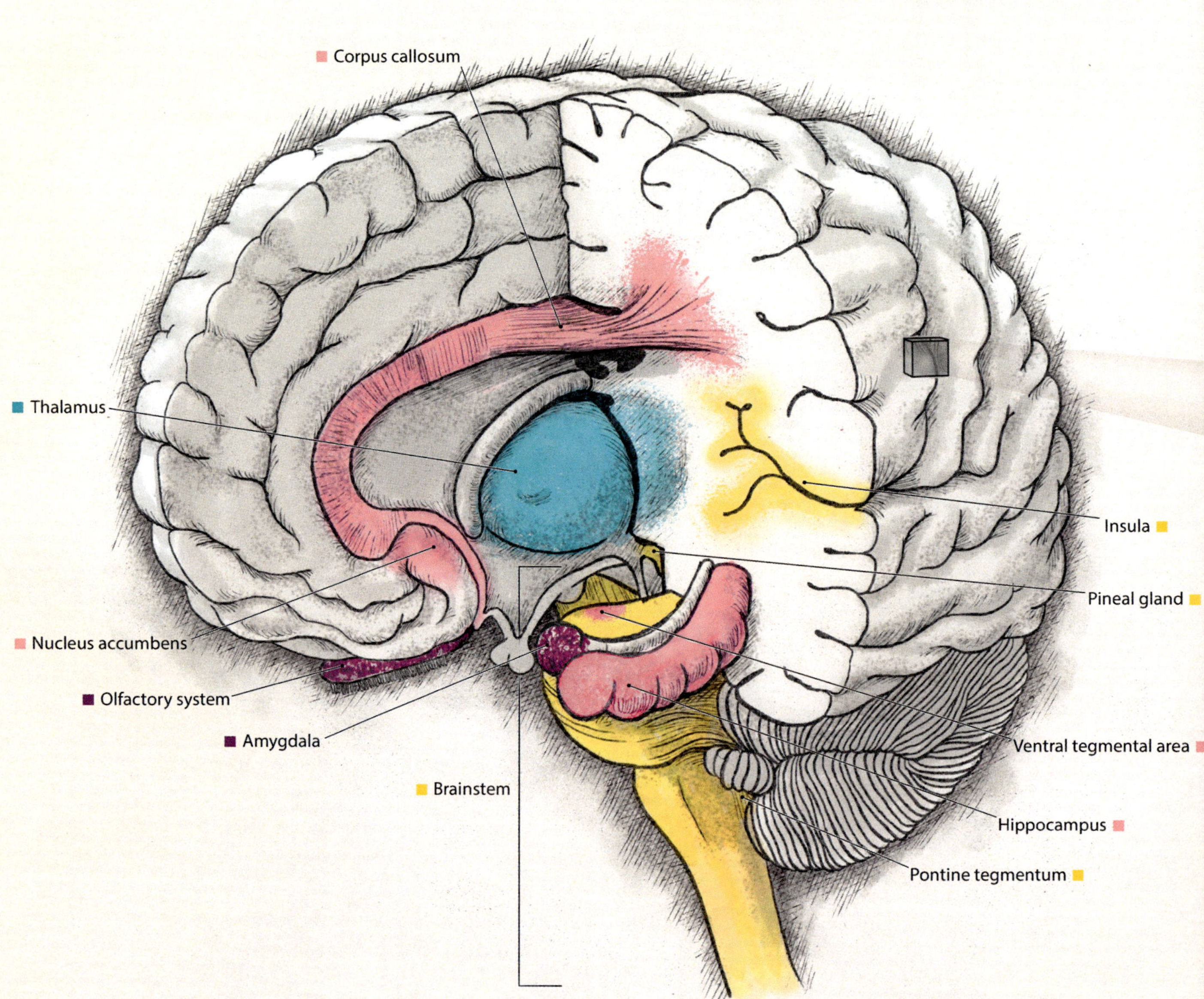

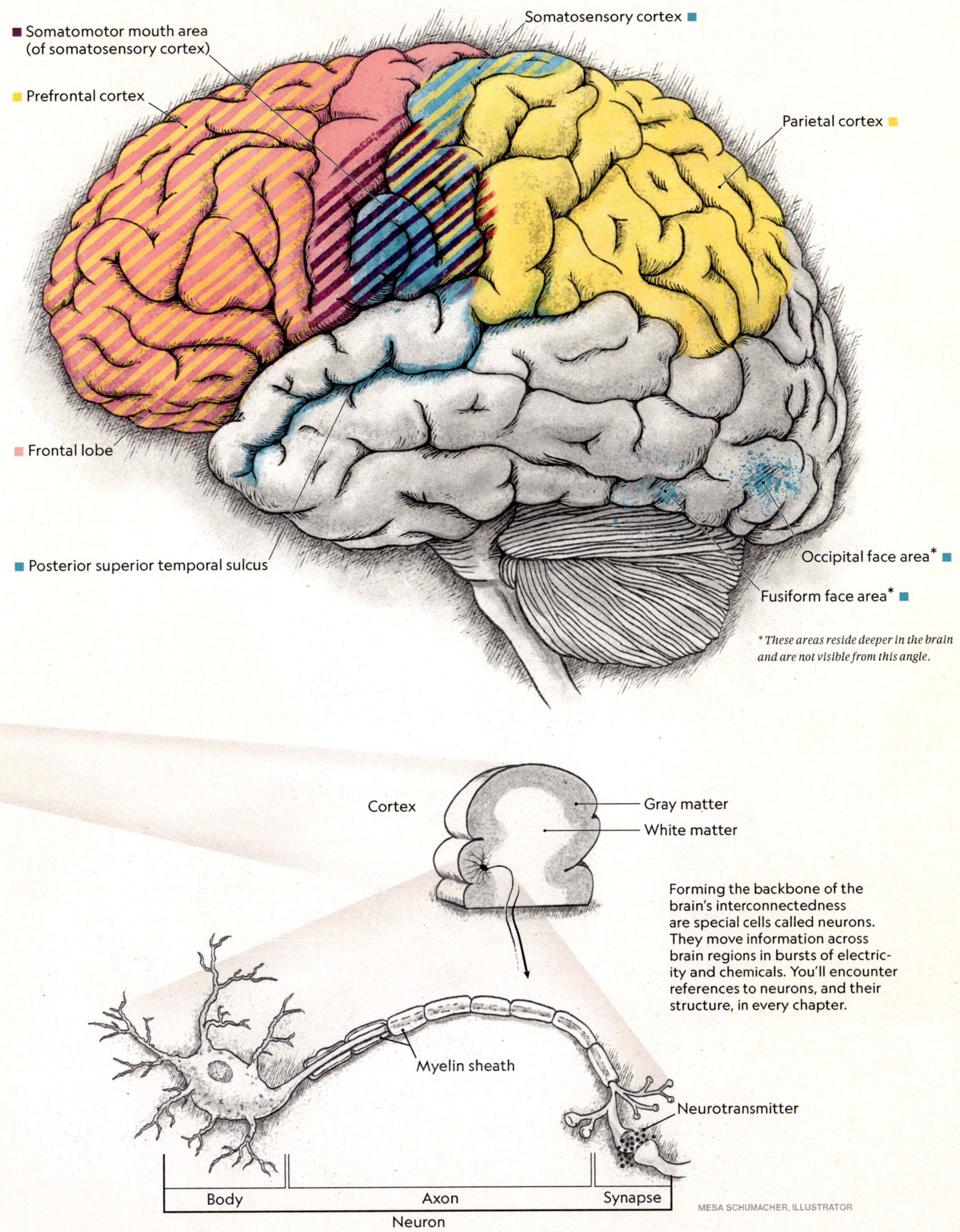

MESA SCHUMACHER, ILLUSTRATOR

CHAPTER 1

YOUR UNIQUE INNER WORLD

Information "highways" connecting different areas of the brain direct how we each perceive the world. Some brains lack a few of these connections, while others have extra.

We each live rich internal lives that others know nothing about. Explaining to someone else how you perceive the world is like trying to describe the color green. It's a hard thing to communicate, and it's easy to assume everyone goes through life the way you do—until someone's innocent question shatters the illusion. "Why are you wearing one red sock and one green sock?" is how many people first figure out they are color blind and others are not.

At the most basic level, humans experience the world through senses—the brain's biologically hardwired reaction to stimuli in the world around us, such as light or sound. Perception is your personal spin on what these sensations mean cognitively. This requires complex interconnection in the brain, leaving room for diverse experiences. Many perceptual differences manifest as benign preferences—one person may love the scent of gasoline, while another will gag—but other differences can dramatically orient the path of a person's life. For some, there are gaps: A lower level of interconnectedness among a brain's face processing regions can lead to prosopagnosia, the inability to recognize faces. For others, there are crosswires: A hyperconnected brain can give rise to synesthesia, in which normally distinct experiences become linked, such as perceiving numbers as having personalities.

People with synesthesia, a neurological experience, have different perceptions of the world—such as tasting shapes. It's common for synesthetes to end up in creative professions. Painter Wassily Kandinsky saw colors when he heard music, and painted this vibrant piece, "Large Study" (detail), in 1914.

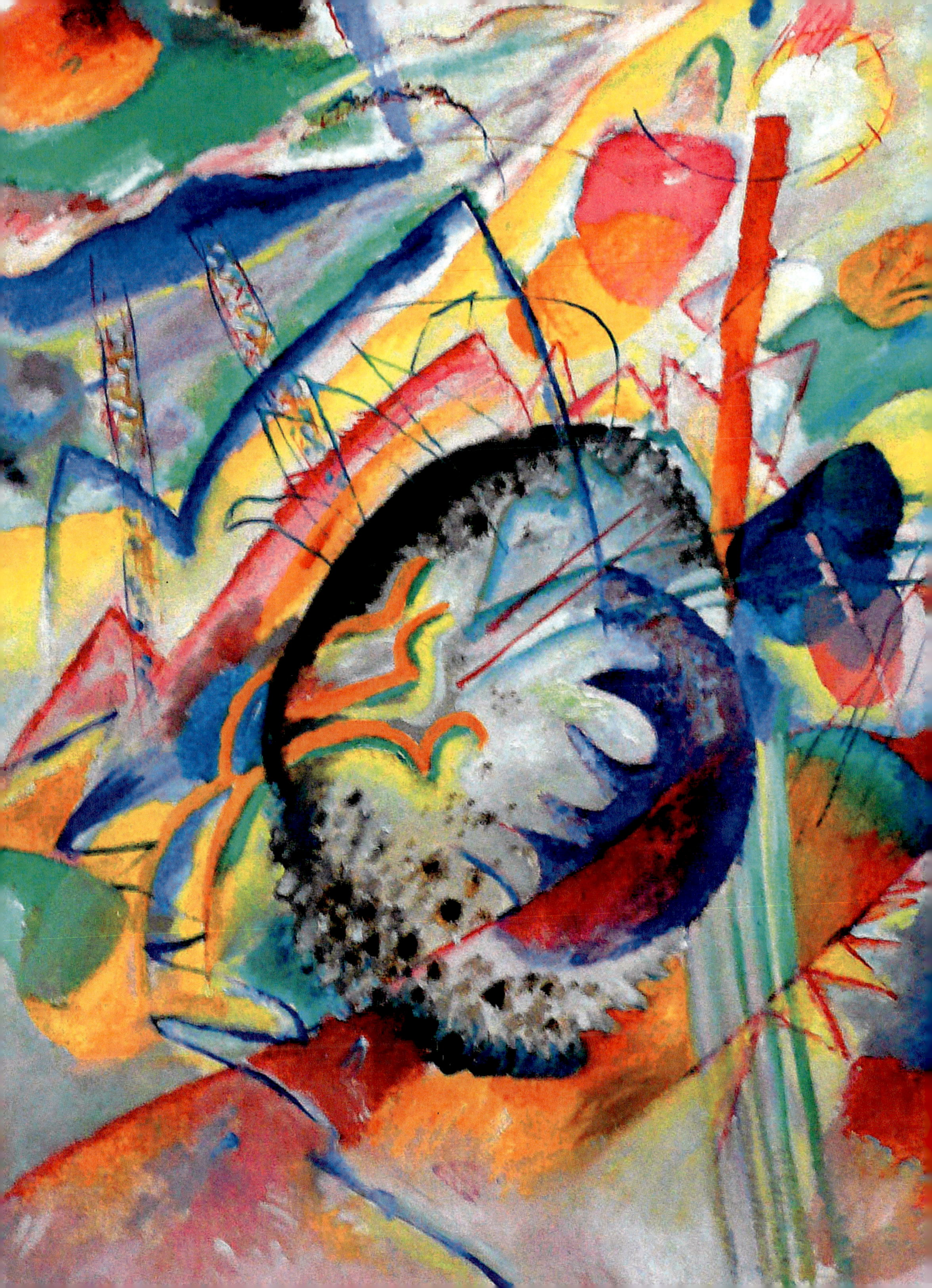

THE FACE OF PROSOPAGNOSIA

FOG ROLLED OVER Lincoln, Nebraska, the morning of the funeral, only breaking under the gentle warmth of the rising June sun. An older man with short, gray hair joined a hundred or so other mourners gathered inside a modern, single-story church. Glasses framed the man's face, and although it was Saturday, he wore his usual Sunday attire: slacks and a button-down. When Ashley Peterson entered the church, she noticed the man and all of these details about him, and panic rose. It was the man they were all here to bury, raised from the dead. Except his presence didn't seem to alarm anyone but her.

Observing a human face is an intimate and uncanny endeavor. You might think you know someone by their features—the exact distribution of colored speckles in their irises, the concave dimple to the left of their smile, or a pronounced freckle on their nose—but the sum of these parts never quite adds up to what makes this face different from a similar one. Yet somehow most people can instantly pick themselves out of a group photograph, or breeze over a room full of strangers at a party to lock eyes with their best friend, the unfamiliar and familiar separating like water and oil. Converting the component parts of a face into something instantly recognizable and memorable is alchemy the human brain is specially designed to do. But not Peterson's.

There were two men at that funeral—one in a coffin, and another very much alive in a pew—who until that moment she never realized were different people. This wasn't simply a laughable mix-up or the consequence of a self-centered, inattentive friend. Peterson's otherwise typical brain is wired to stall out when confronted with faces, a disorder called developmental prosopagnosia. The name comes from the Greek words for "face" and "non-knowledge," and it's a lifelong experience that occurs from birth.

"I felt a bit like an imposter at the funeral," says Peterson, a 38-year-old special education teacher. "Did I ever know that man? Did I even deserve to be there? And I felt a bit guilty that I was glad the man I thought was dead was still alive, when everyone else was grieving."

WHEN SHE MEETS someone, Peterson can get as far as noting their facial features as simple facts about them, but she can't meaningfully grasp or hang onto the gestalt of what she sees. She's not visually impaired—she can perceive your eyes, your nose, and more—but as soon as she blinks or walks away, the image vanishes, even while she may remember a fact, such as eye color. She sometimes writes notes for herself about people she's supposed to know, such as her boss ("wears hair in bun"), but if they change anything about their appearance, Peterson is lost. Or, as in the case of the two men from church, if they share a similar appearance, she'll never know the difference. The men at her church were about the same age, wore the same clothes and glasses, and had the same hair—they even had the same name. She likens her experience with recognizing faces to

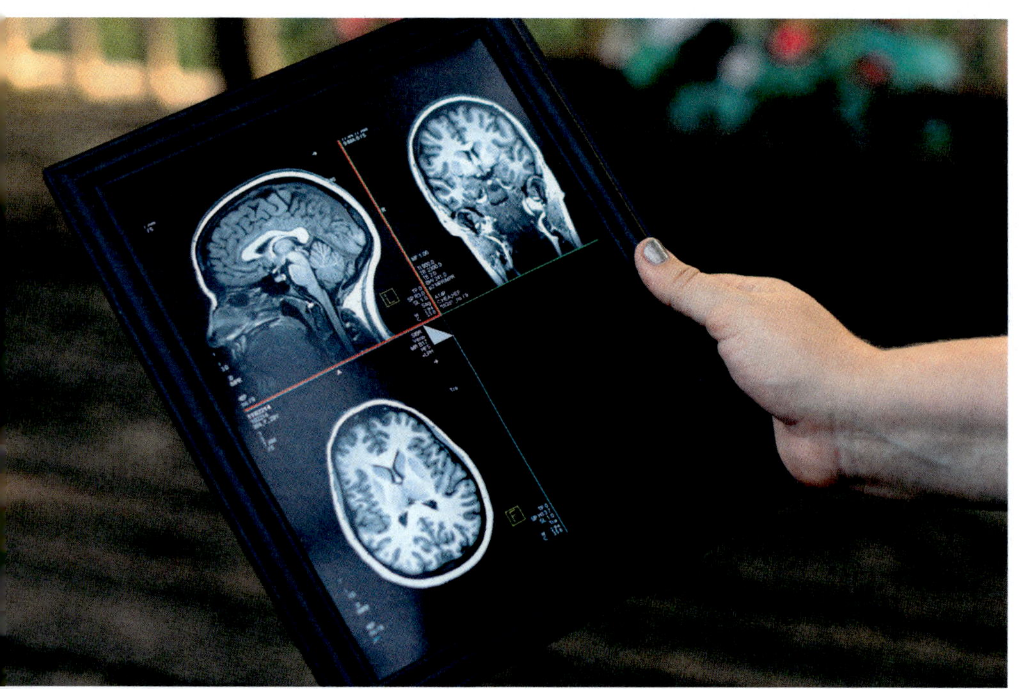

In her home in Lincoln, Nebraska, Ashley Peterson displays a scan of her brain, a souvenir from a study she participated in at Carnegie Mellon University's Behrmann Lab.

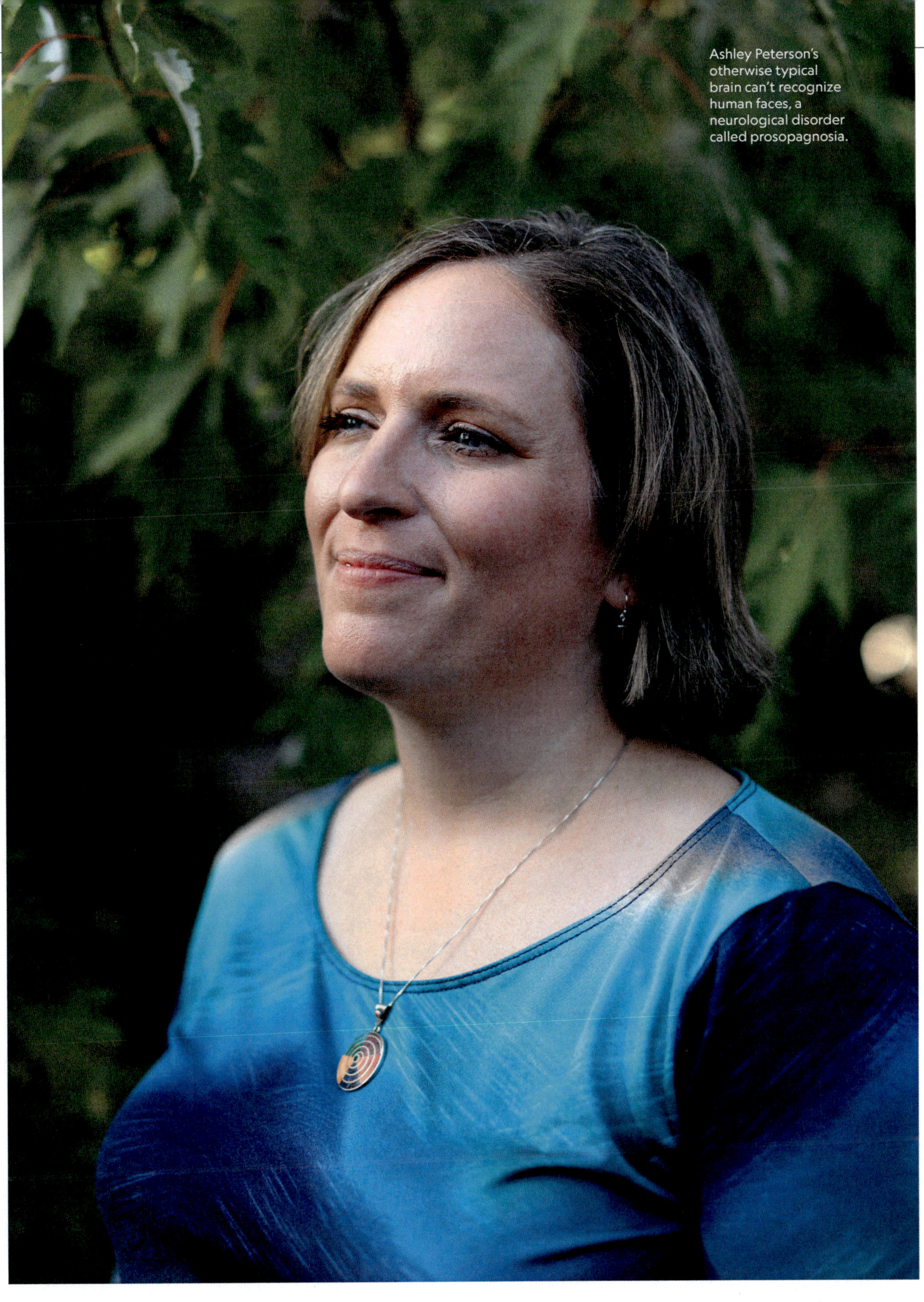
Ashley Peterson's otherwise typical brain can't recognize human faces, a neurological disorder called prosopagnosia.

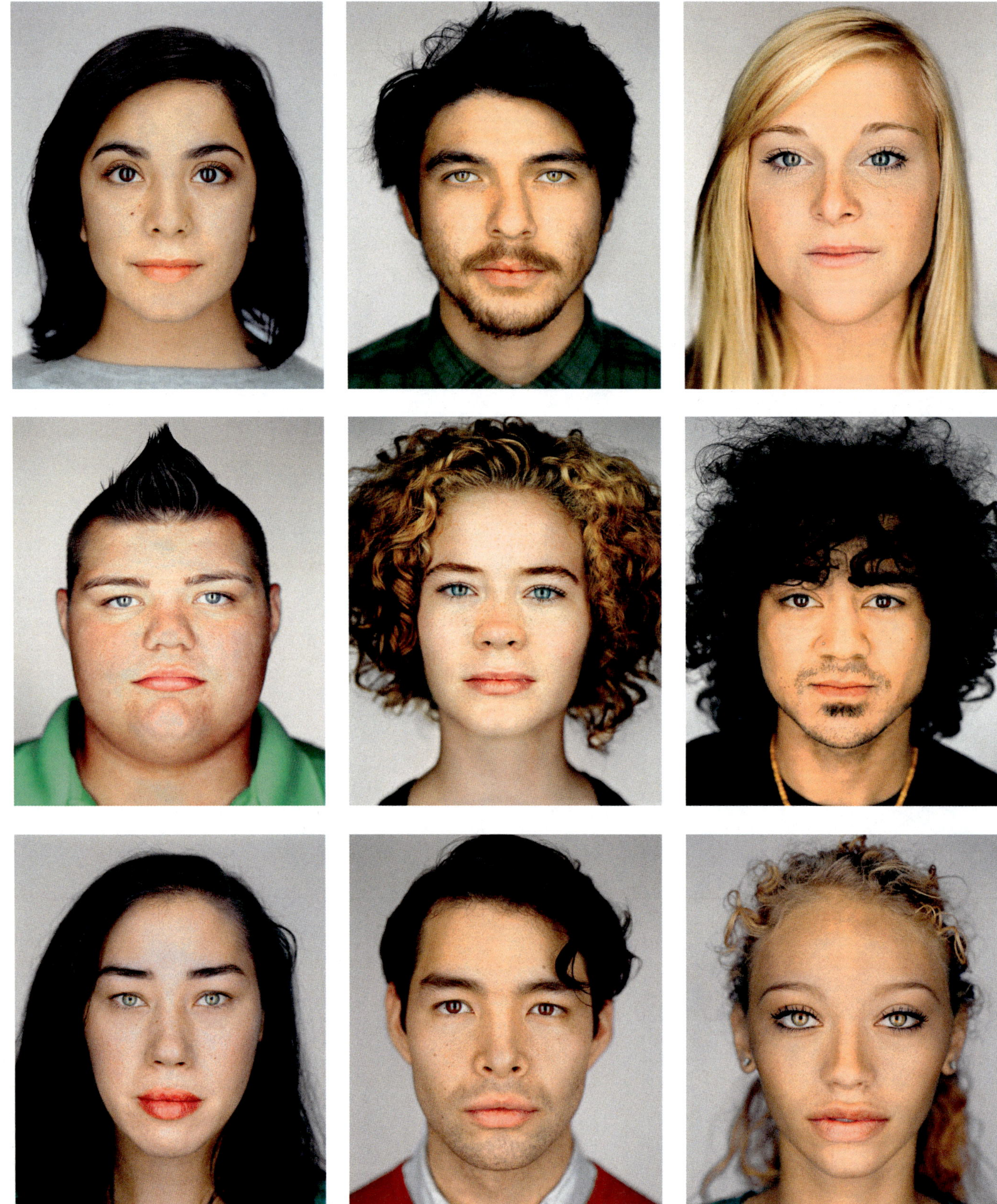

studying an oak leaf, then throwing the leaf back into a pile of 1,000 oak leaves; she'll never find the original again. Growing up, she loved watching *Star Trek* because the characters wear never-changing, color-coded uniforms (she finds television shows and movies with large casts otherwise difficult to follow).

With negligible training, most people find individual, recurring human faces marvelously knowable in a way that far surpasses recognition of other objects and patterns. The average brain can store data for 5,000 faces at any one time, but this feat is nearly impossible for as many as one in every 50 people in the world born with the same disorder as Peterson. A much tinier fraction, about 1 in 30,000, have what's called acquired prosopagnosia, something that arises later in life from brain injury or stroke. Neurologist Joachim Bodamer first described prosopagnosia in the brains of injured World War II veterans in 1947. And Helen McConachie, a clinical psychologist, detailed the developmental variation in a case report 29 years later.

Imagine the feeling of running into a coworker at a grocery store, out of

In lieu of recognizing whole faces, people with prosopagnosia often compensate by memorizing hairstyles, a distinctive mole, or even the sound of someone's voice.

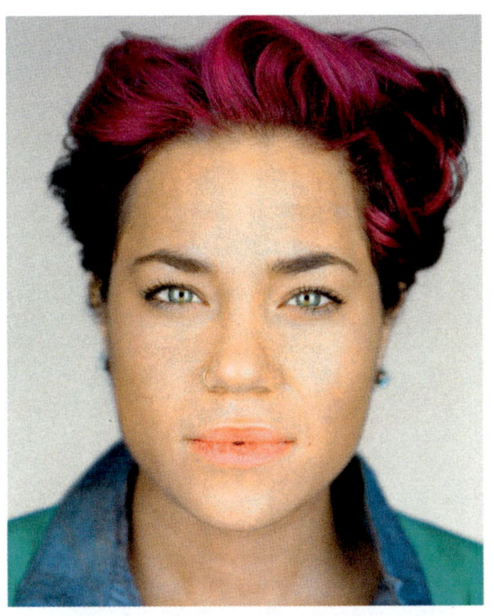

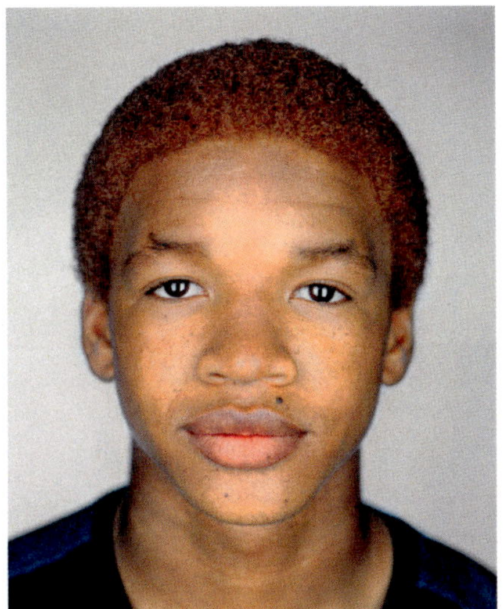

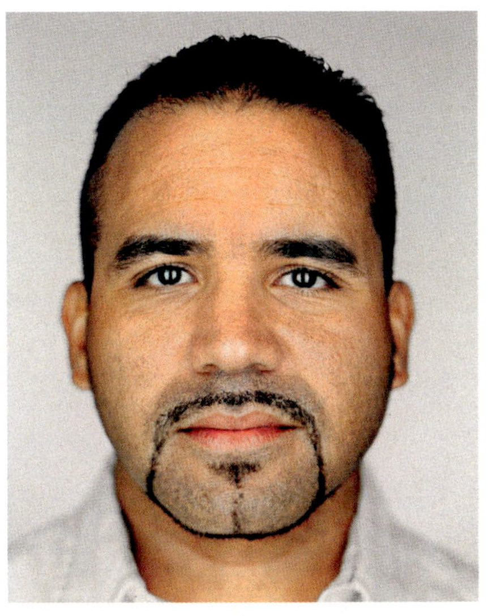

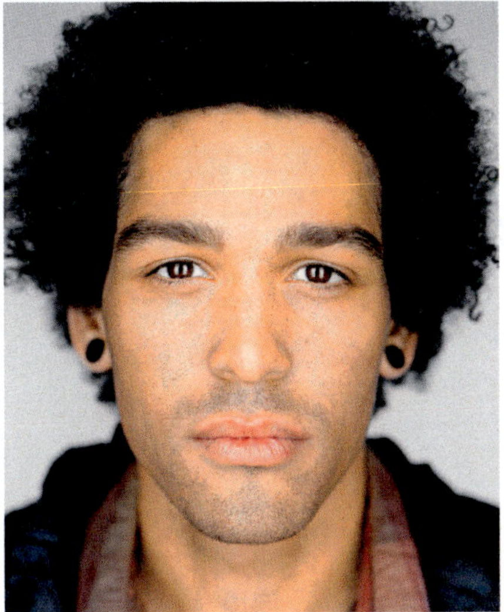

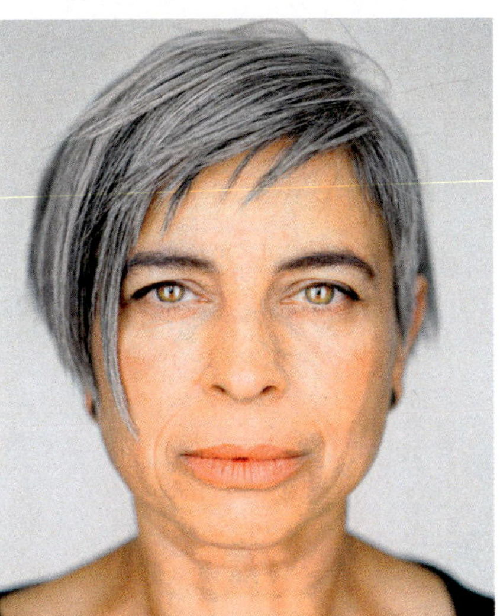

Observing a human face is an intimate and uncanny endeavor. You might think you know someone by their features . . . but the sum of these parts never quite adds up to what makes this face different from a similar one.

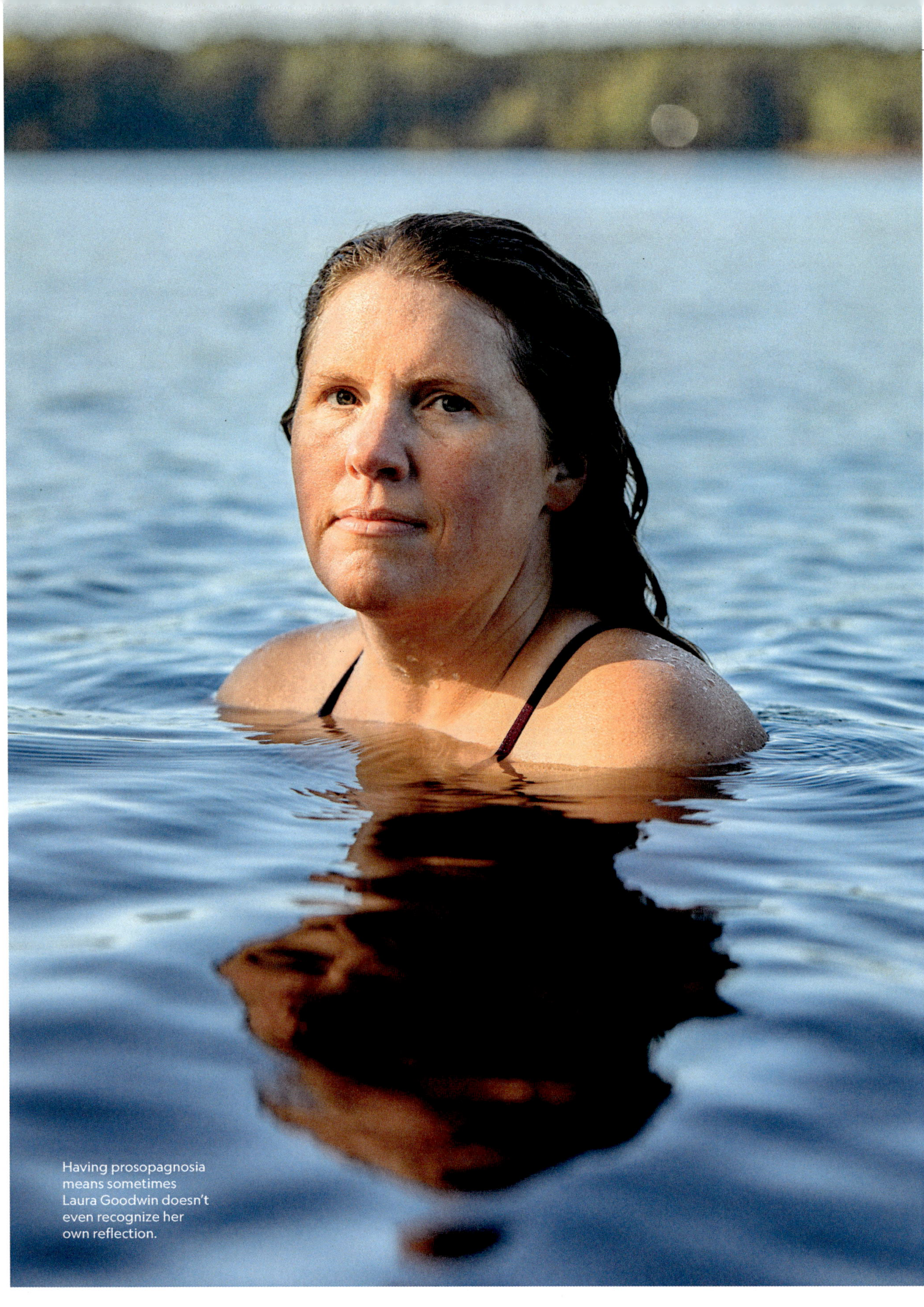

Having prosopagnosia means sometimes Laura Goodwin doesn't even recognize her own reflection.

context, and having that moment of terror when someone you can't place seems to know you. Now imagine having this feeling constantly. It's no wonder so many prosopagnosics end up developing their own clever ways of navigating a planet with 7.9 billion facial strangers, some of whom may even live in their home.

MEMORY MISFIRES

LAURA GOODWIN GLIMPSES a woman nearby while in a department store. They're both standing still, surrounded by racks of clothes they're considering. It's only when Goodwin and the woman begin to move in sync that she realizes she's caught her own reflection in a four-sided, floor-to-ceiling mirror, and mistaken herself for someone else—again. "It's as easy for me to misrecognize myself as it is to misrecognize other people," she says.

Goodwin, a 44-year-old swim coach, didn't realize this wasn't everyday life for other people until graduate school, when a friend came home from a seminar on prosopagnosia and told Goodwin about the disorder. Goodwin immediately felt sure she had it. "I didn't even realize how well other people could [recognize faces]," she says. "You always think your lived experience is what everyone's experience is like."

Joe DeGutis, who researches prosopagnosia at the VA Boston Healthcare System and Harvard University, finds that many participants in his studies thought they were just lazy or inattentive. Receiving a diagnosis sometimes makes people want to reassess their whole childhood. "It's a little bit of a stealth disorder," he says.

Prosopagnosia is sometimes colloquially referred to as "face blindness," but that's a misnomer, as it's not a malfunction of the basic visual sense. Researchers primarily understand it as a disorder of visual perception, in that a person can see component parts of something without perceiving the whole entity.

But new research suggests that some types of prosopagnosia may be something outside the realm of vision entirely: a subtype of the disorder arises when memory misfires.

SEEING FACES EVERYWHERE

If you've ever glanced at a North American electrical outlet and seen the socket holes as an alarmed face, that's because the human brain is evolutionarily predisposed to find faces in everyday objects. The sensation, called face pareidolia, is so strong it can even give rise to feelings of empathy, fear, or humor—even while on some level we know we're looking at an inanimate object.

Although human faces vary greatly in their details, they're very similar in terms of the placement of eyes, nose, and mouth. Objects with similar distributions of features seem to trigger our face recognition system. A network of brain areas is specially trained to identify the pattern of human faces and is so attuned to its job that it sometimes overachieves.

Researchers at the University of New South Wales in Sydney, Australia, found the overly sensitive facial recognition system at the core of face pareidolia by testing sensory adaptation, an illusion in which repeatedly being shown similar prompts can change a person's perception. If someone is shown pictures of faces with eyes looking left again and again, when they finally see a different picture, one with a face with eyes gazing straight ahead, they'll perceive the gaze as looking to the right. To test the perceptual systems at play in face pareidolia, researchers slipped some face-like, nonhuman pictures into the batch and still saw the sensory adaptation effect, as though they had used pictures of human faces. This implies the brain wasn't processing these inanimate faces any differently. This overzealous recognition may be an evolutionary device to help promote social interactions as much as possible.

A NETWORK OF INFORMATION

TO INSTANTLY RECOGNIZE familiar faces, the brain typically taps into a complex internal network of a few different areas that really seem to prefer faces over other objects. The occipital face area focuses on component parts of a face, while the posterior superior temporal sulcus handles the dynamic aspects of a face, such as where someone's eyes are looking or if they're expressing an emotion. The fusiform face area brings it all together into a meaningful whole.

Those who acquire prosopagnosia following a brain injury may be missing areas of the brain crucial to this network. Those born with prosopagnosia have all the brain areas in this network, and they're functioning, it's just the communication among them that's fractured. It's like having a computer powered up and the URL for a website typed in, but the page won't load because the fiber optic cables that carry internet signals are down.

Prosopagnosia is sometimes colloquially referred to as "face blindness," but that's a misnomer, as it's not a malfunction of the basic visual sense.

Central to the networks in your brain are neurons, nerve cells which transmit information. To communicate with each other, neurons release and receive chemicals called neurotransmitters. The signal to release these chemicals, or a response to receiving them, is electricity that moves up and down a neuron's axon. The axon is a trunk-like structure connecting a neuron's cell body (which generates the electricity) and its dendrites, the branches that release neurotransmitters. It would take too long for electricity to move along the whole of every axon in the brain so, to speed up communication, axons typically come wrapped in intermittent sheaths of protein and fat called myelin that allow electrical impulses to jump like stones skipping water.

Clusters of neuronal cell bodies make up the brain's famous gray matter where information is processed, but the axons make up the brain's equally

What some prosopagnosics are really struggling with when they can't recognize faces is associating them with contextual information. Memory training can help.

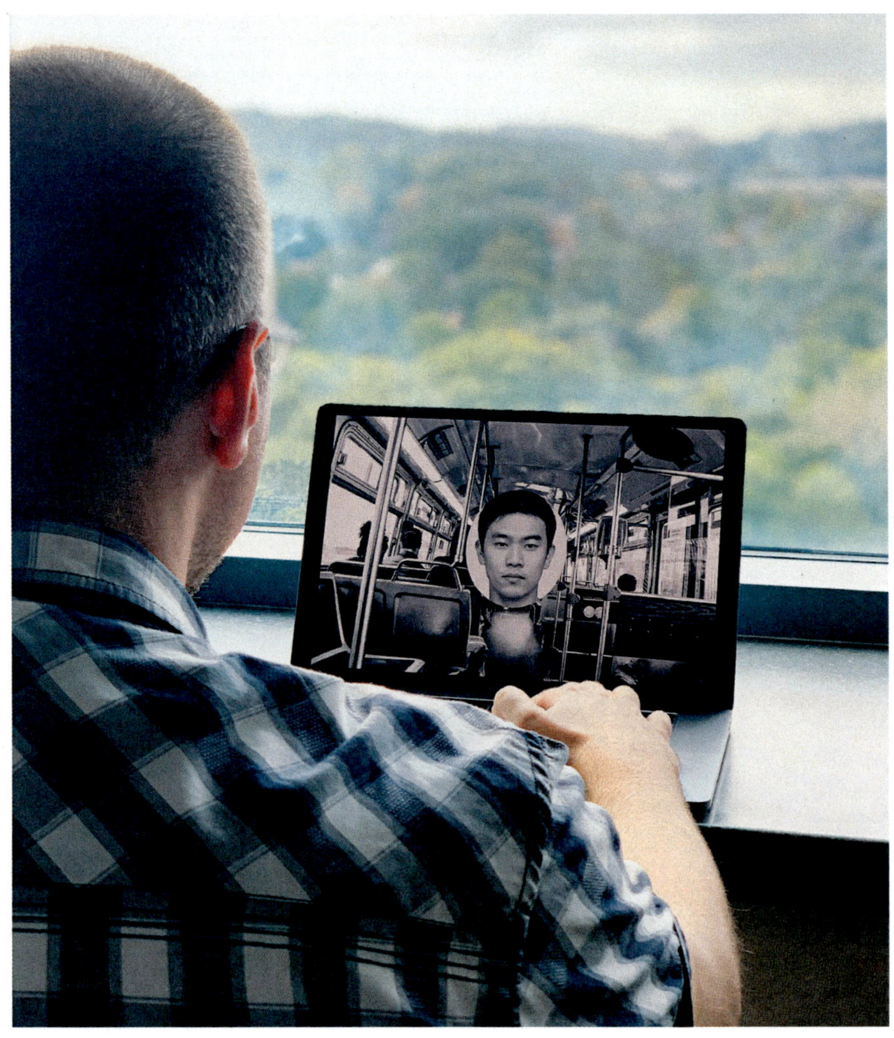

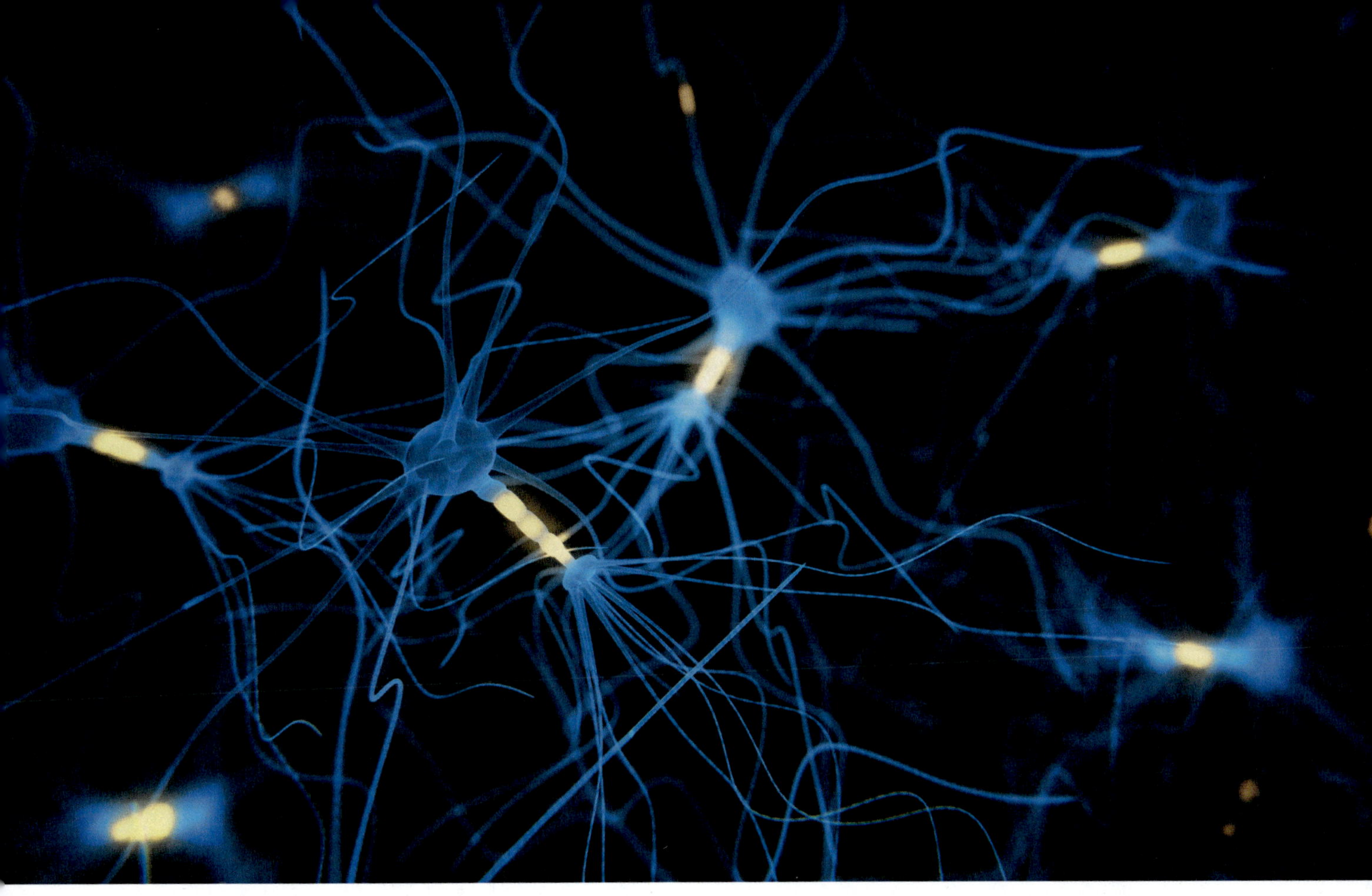

Myelin sheaths (shown in yellow) wrap typical neurons in protein and fat, helping electricity—and thus information—move quickly. Some prosopagnosic brains lack this feature.

vital white matter, where information is transferred. A group of naked axons without their myelin sheaths can slow a system of information exchange from a sprint to a crawl, which is what DeGutis sees in the cells connecting face recognition areas in prosopagnosics' brains. "Does that mean you can put someone in a scanner and just say immediately they're prosopagnosic? No, we're not quite there yet," DeGutis says. But the first time he and his team noticed this structural difference, "it was pretty dramatic that this whole network, and the connections between these nodes, was just ramped down."

One thing that continued to confound DeGutis after this discovery was that some prosopagnosics do score perfectly fine on general visual perception assessments, failing only to recognize faces. This challenged the definition of prosopagnosia as a visual perception disorder. Assuming there was something else going on, DeGutis developed more sophisticated diagnostics, and he found that some prosopagnosics may actually be struggling with what can be better described as a memory disorder. It's true that some prosopagnosics can neither recall faces they've seen before nor can they tease apart two different side-by-side faces as being distinct. But others *can* tell the side-by-sides apart, it's just that a few seconds later they can't pick out which faces they've already seen. For the latter group, their issue is with recollection, not familiarity.

DIAGNOSING PROSOPAGNOSIA WITH more specificity paves the way for experimental cognitive training. Prosopagnosia is a historically incurable disorder with major social ramifications, but prosopagnosics who struggle with memory have a chance at improving their facial recognition prowess with practice. DeGutis and his lab designed sessions to train prosopagnosics to link someone's face with other attributes—the person's occupation, or even an assumption about them, such as whether a person comes across as introverted or extroverted. Most people do a bit of this automatically, and super-recognizers do it exceptionally well.

Goodwin, the woman who hasn't always recognized herself in a mirror, sees a change in her abilities from participating in the training sessions and is considering how she might share these tools with one of her young sons,

CLOSER LOOK

THE FORGOTTEN SIXTH SENSE

Sight, smell, taste, hearing, and touch are always in the sensory spotlight, but another key sense for navigating the world is your brain's knowledge of where your body is at all times.

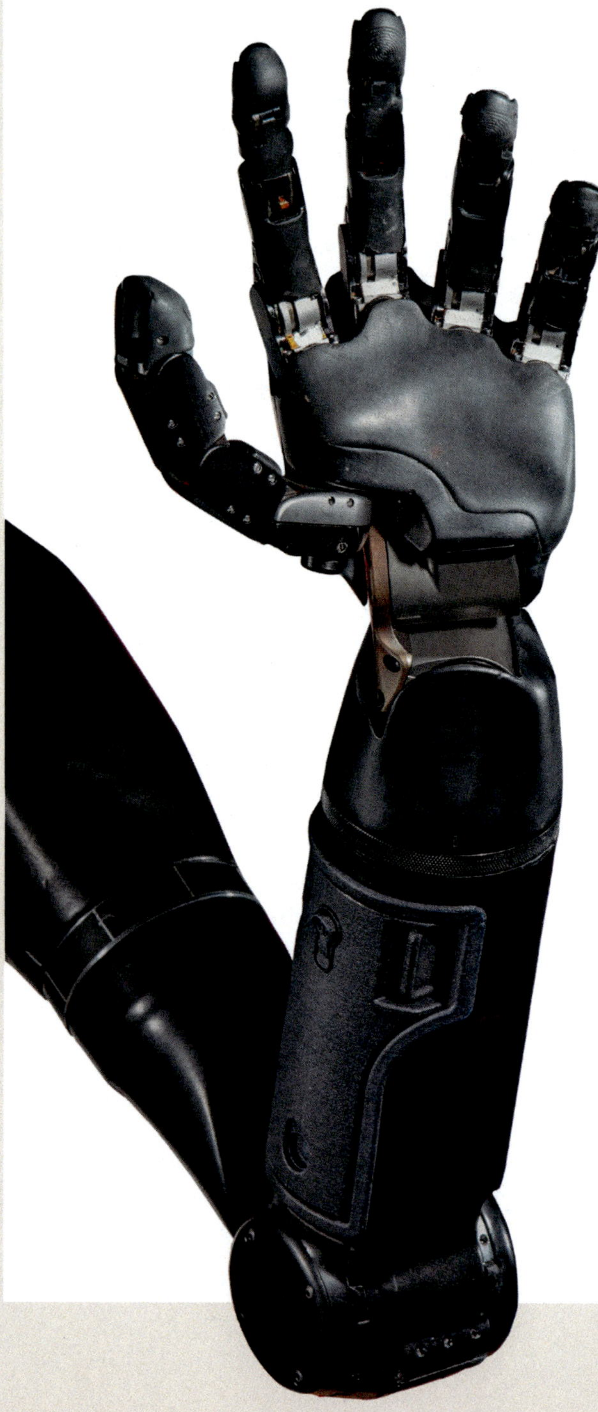

Put your hands at your sides and close your eyes. Then, touch your nose with your right pointer finger. You probably did this with ease, but this action would've been impossible without a covert sensory system the brain operates every time you move. Proprioception is your ability to know the exact position, speed, and rotation of all parts of your body without conscious effort. While you may not think of this as a sensory experience in the way that vision or hearing loom large, life would be quite difficult without it.

Electrical Highways

All over the body, and at every joint especially, clusters of neurons send information back to the brain along electrical highways—the tubular parts of the cell called axons. Each of these electrical impulses rapidly informs the brain of the specific position of, say, your wrist. A surface-level area at the top of the brain, called the somatosensory cortex, then calculates the geometric adjustments necessary to land your finger exactly on your nose. It's a small miracle that you can do this effortlessly. "Sometimes it's given the moniker 'the sixth sense,'" says Krishna Shenoy, director of the Neural Prosthetic Systems Lab at Stanford University. "The reason for that is you're not sensing something external to the body, you're sensing something internal to the body, and we just take it for granted. We don't even think about it, we just use it."

Next-generation prosthetic limbs can interact with the brain, but are still missing proprioception, a key internal sense of the body's location.

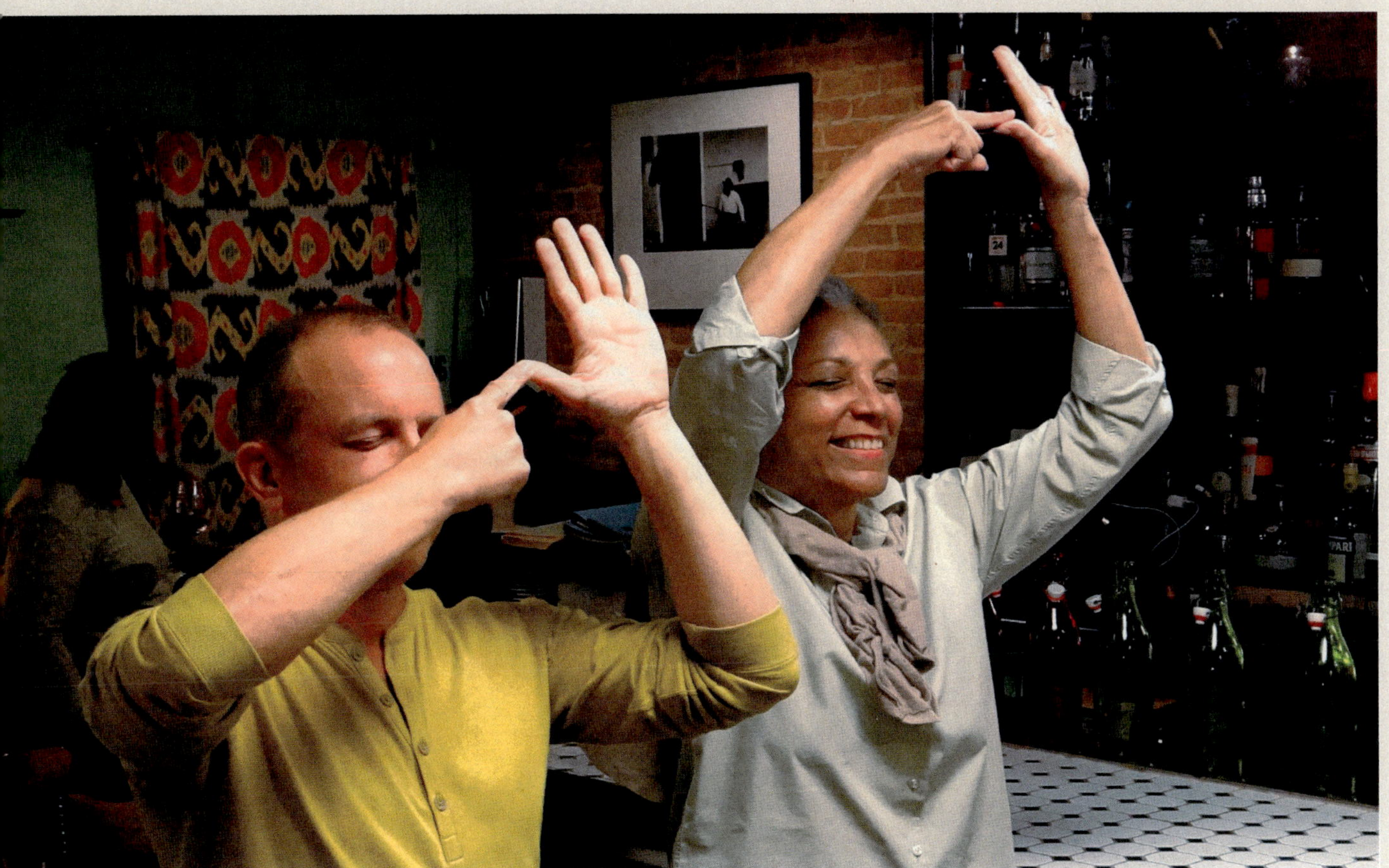

One way to test your own sense of proprioception is by closing your eyes, holding your left hand out in front of you, and moving your right pointer finger from your left thumb, to your nose, and back again.

Navigating the World

This special system is far more efficient than using vision to do the same job. While seeing can feel like a seamless movie, vision is actually pretty slow and ill-suited for helping you move through the world on its own, compared to proprioception. It takes about 100 to 150 milliseconds from the time light hits your eye to when your brain sorts out what's going on; proprioception, on the other hand, happens within five milliseconds. "It's radically faster," says Shenoy.

The incredible speed of proprioception is critical to having control over your body. While some may struggle with balance or motor coordination, it's incredibly rare for someone to be completely missing their proprioceptive sense. Those who are will be able to take only a few steps blindfolded before falling over, and they can't reach out and find an object they were just looking at if their eyes are closed. They have to rely primarily on the imperfect visual system to make up for their lack of proprioception.

How people navigate the world with artificial limbs is a more common proprioceptive concern. Watch someone with a prosthetic hand move to pick something up off a counter and you'll notice they'll grip the item slowly—that's because they're also relying entirely on vision, with a broken feedback loop between the hand and the brain.

Increasingly sophisticated robotics can close part of this loop by sending impulses from the brain to a prosthetic hand, causing it to move. But without a way to return impulses back to the brain, it's very difficult to do things most of us take for granted, such as the nose-touching exercise, with your eyes shut. Clinical trials are currently underway to test prosthetics that can offer true proprioception to the wearer, completing the circle of communication from limb to brain, and back again.

who she suspects may also have prosopagnosia. It's a disorder that likely runs in families. But not all prosopagnosics will benefit from the training, and not all prosopagnosics want to. Peterson, the woman in Nebraska, feels her "proso," as she calls the disorder, is a unique part of who she is, something crucial to her open-mindedness.

"I really have a hard time telling who is attractive or not," she says. "Instead, what ends up being attractive to me is someone's personality . . . One of the benefits to my proso is that it really forces me to get to know a person, and not rely on physical appearance or these first impressions."

But she has some tough moments. Peterson used to be able to easily tell her nieces apart by their height, but now that they're teenagers, she's not only mixing them up with each other but also not recognizing them out in public. On a recent family bike ride, Peterson stopped to help her nephew fix his wheel while her nieces went ahead. When one niece came back to check on them, Peterson thought she was a stranger asking if they needed help and waved her off.

"When I finally realized who she was, it just hit so hard," says Peterson.

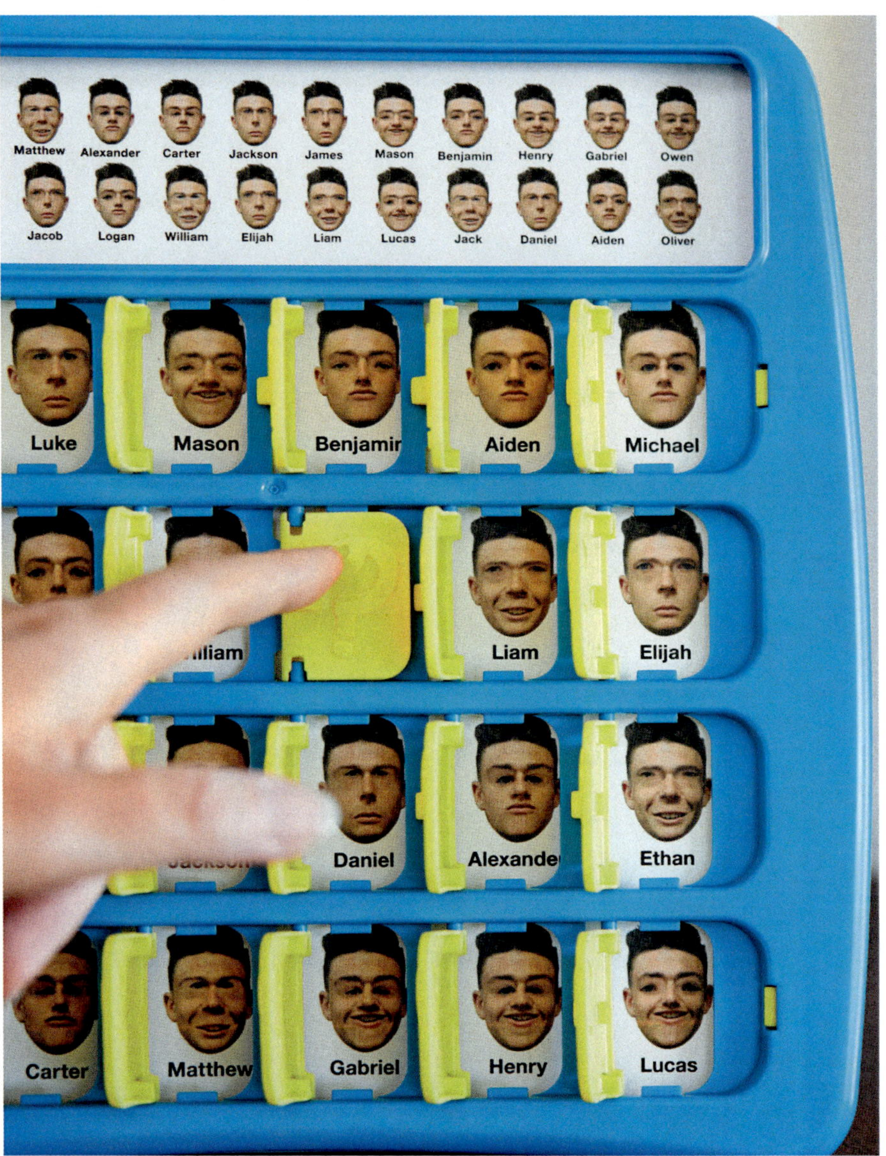

Laura Goodwin uses a series of increasingly difficult games of *Guess Who* that scientists have modified to try and train her brain to recognize faces.

To instantly recognize familiar faces, the brain typically taps into a complex internal network of a few different areas that really seem to prefer faces over other objects.

"This person that you love, and that you care for—to not be able to recognize them, to see them as a stranger, that was so hard for me."

Still, even without the typical perceptual—or memory—capacity that most others have when it comes to faces, people with prosopagnosia like Peterson and Goodwin color their worlds by intimately knowing the voices of all their friends or being especially open-minded when meeting new people. Experiencing the world differently from the status quo is something they also share with a group of people whose lives are the opposite: brimming with extra perceptual abilities.

THE LANGUAGE OF SYNESTHESIA

WHEN MARY BICHNER composes music, she's transcribing the auditory language of the colors around her, something most people's brains can't do. On a scorching July day at Mount Auburn Cemetery in Cambridge, Massachusetts, the two of us met and sought shade on the stone steps of an old chapel, where she showed me how her favorite chord, E-flat major, was hovering nearby. She pointed to her dress, a jewel-tone blue, the plentiful green foliage around us, and finally, to a refreshing shock of orange flowers poking out of the ground to our right. From 2016 to 2017, she was the composer-in-residence here, the first garden cemetery in the United States, composing suites of music based on the collective hues of the resplendent landscaping and waterways, active wildlife, and stained-glass sanctuaries. The environment was ideal for a brain delighted by color.

Bichner has synesthesia, an automatic perceptual ability that fills a person's world with extra information most people don't experience. What synesthetes and prosopagnosics share is having no idea they experience life differently from other people until someone else points it out.

In high school, a friend inquired how Bichner, who has perfect pitch, recognized notes without flaw or hesitation. "I said, 'Oh, you know, if I think of F, I see purple,'" Bichner recalls. "That was the first time I was kind of aware of it." But she didn't learn what this sound-color experience was until her early 20s, when she visited a message board for fans of the rock band Radiohead. People described the colors they saw when listening to the music and called it synesthesia. The internet age has been a major catalyst in people's awareness of their different perceptual abilities, and in finding others who share them. Message boards and social media groups have been similarly illuminating for prosopagnosics and people with other so-called disorders, and researchers increasingly use these online communities to connect with them.

During her residency, the two six-song suites Bichner composed came from the most vibrant seasons in the cemetery, autumn and spring. One day, she walked to the top of Washington Tower, a lookout from the 1850s with a panoramic view of the Greater Boston area, and found one of her more unusual color combinations in the wild: the fall foliage had turned to orange, the grass was green, and one single purple flower was still hanging on from summer. "For this one song, I was so happy because I really wanted it to be in B flat, and those are the colors," she says. "I was always pleasantly surprised to find my color combinations."

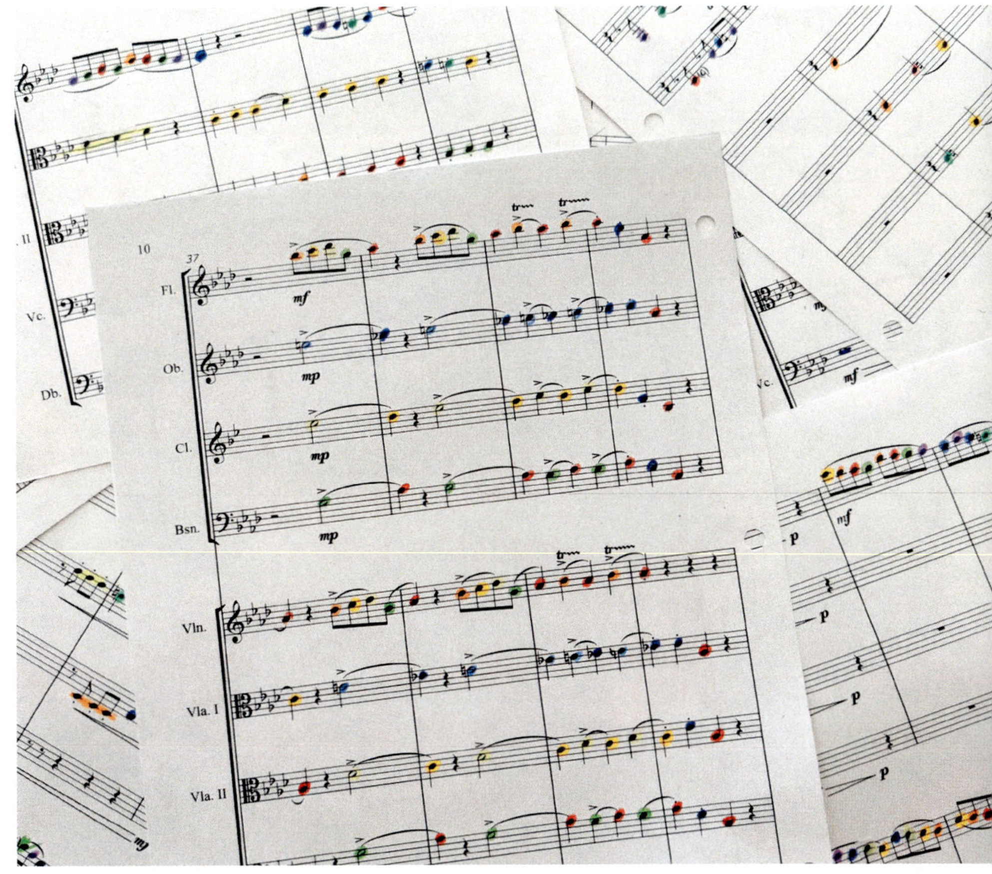

Mary Bichner's color-coded score for *Allegro Moderato in Ab [Autumn Suite]*, a suite she composed based on autumnal hues. Her synesthetic brain can hear colors.

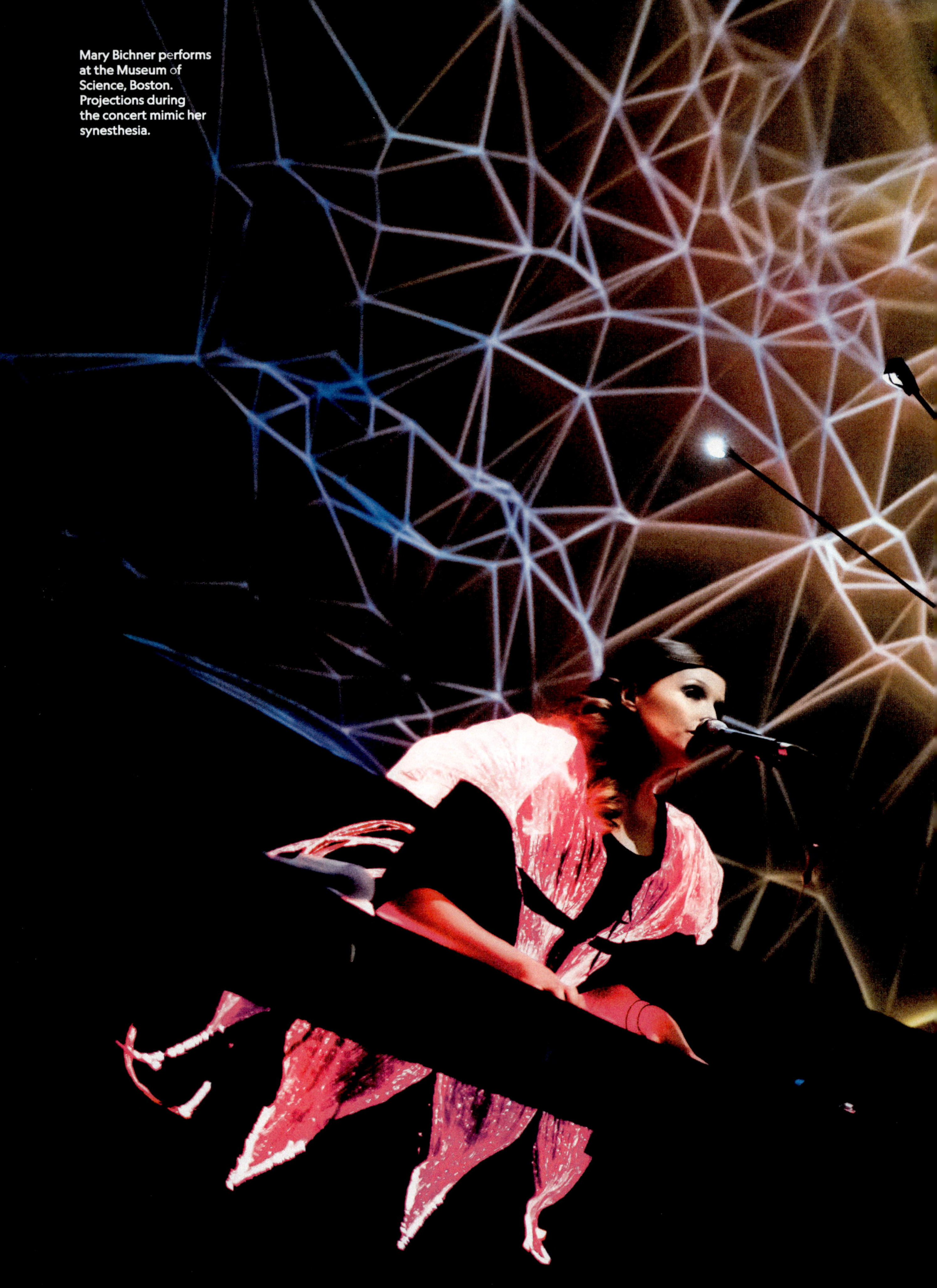

Mary Bichner performs at the Museum of Science, Boston. Projections during the concert mimic her synesthesia.

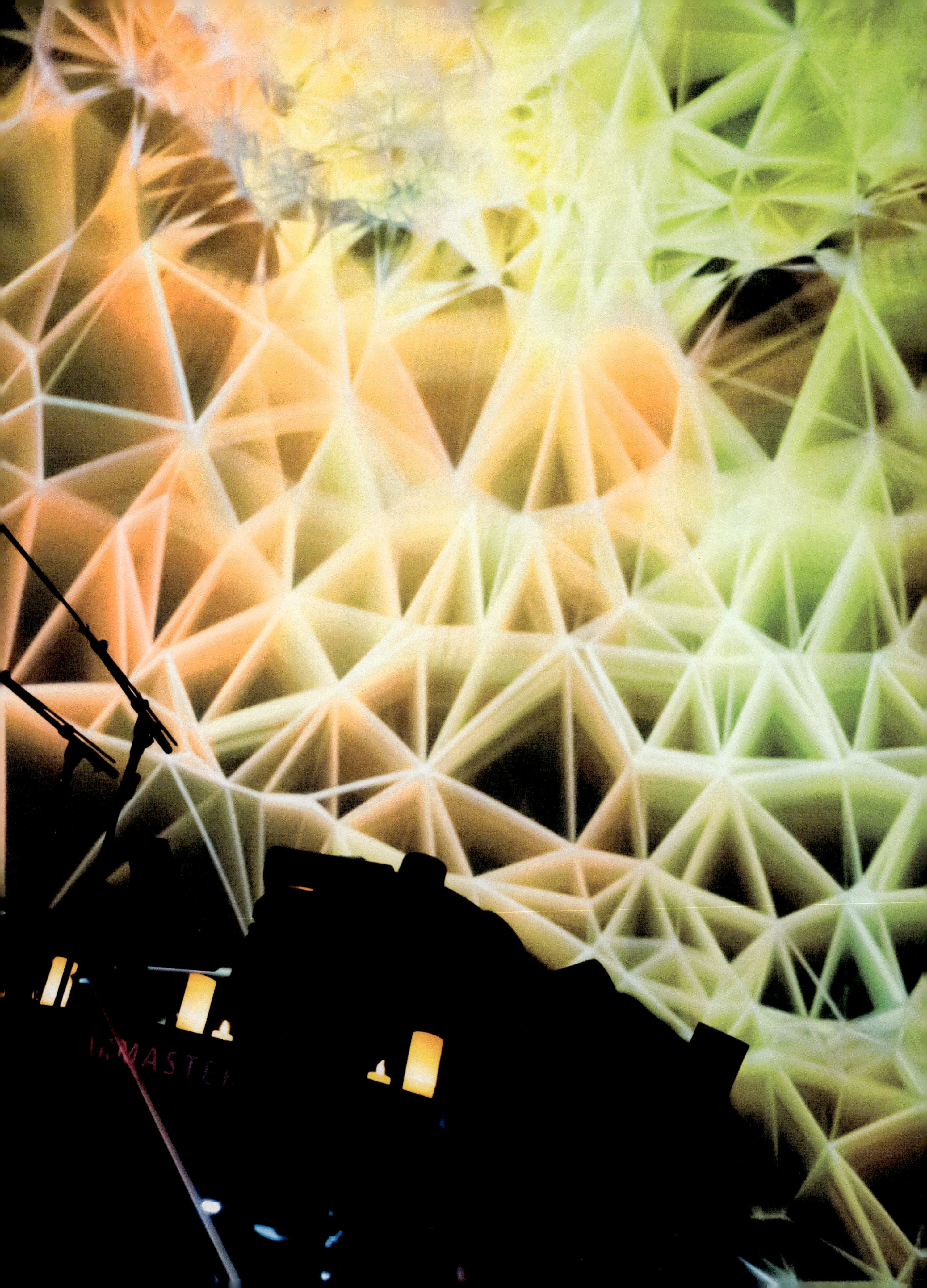

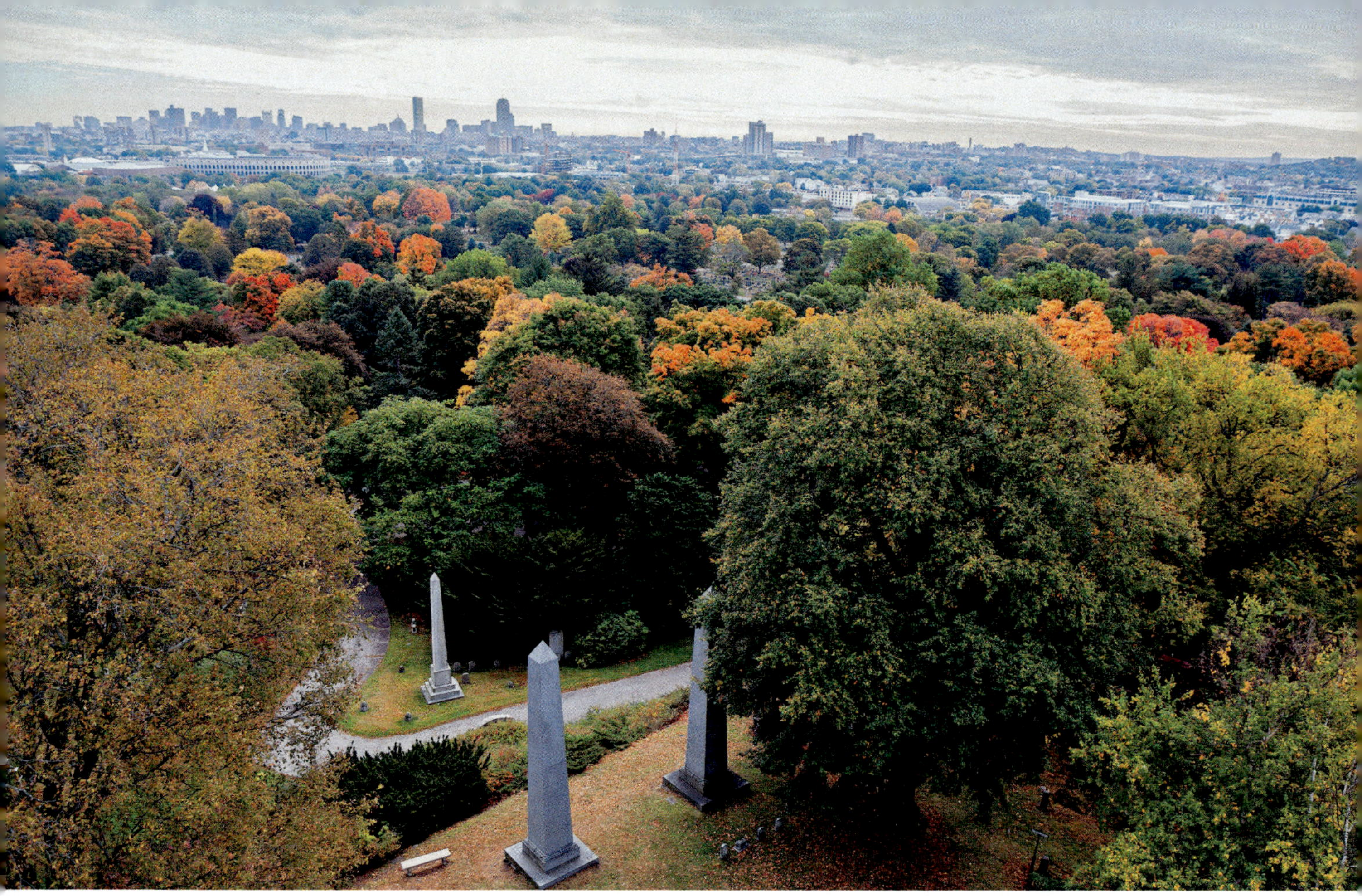

Downtown Boston as seen from Mount Auburn Cemetery. The garden cemetery offered vibrant, seasonal inspiration to composer Mary Bichner, who hears colors. *Left:* Mary Bichner labeled colored pencils to show the note she hears upon seeing each.

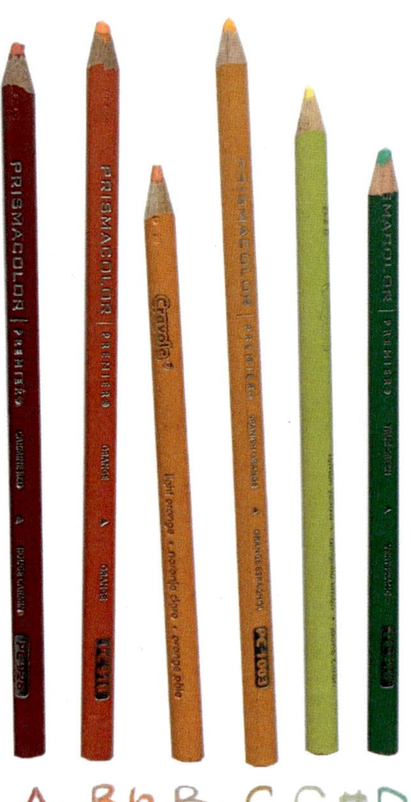

MORE THAN MERGING THE SENSES

LAYPEOPLE, SCIENTISTS, AND even synesthetes themselves commonly describe these perceptual experiences as a merging of the senses. Something that allows them to have what to others seem like fantastical, impossible experiences—such as tasting the sound of a person's voice or, as with Mary Bichner, hearing colors. Historically, synesthesia has been labeled a sensory disorder. But new research is challenging this, redefining synesthesia as an experience, not a disorder, and one not strictly of the sensorial variety.

"A pure definition is of limited use if it doesn't capture the full spectrum of manifestation," says Julia Simner, a neuropsychologist who runs the MULTISENSE lab at the University of Sussex in England. "Continuing to insist that synesthesia has to involve the senses would exclude some of the really widely accepted [types]."

She's referring to grapheme-color synesthesia, in which people perceive black letters and numbers on a white background (monochrome graphemes) to have consistent colors that appear to them either directly on the page or in their mind's eye. Even just thinking about a letter or number can trigger an internal sense of the associated color. But this isn't, strictly speaking, a mash-up of two sensory experiences, like hearing and seeing or hearing and tasting—grapheme-color synesthesia is really about concepts, not senses.

IN 2006, EDWARD HUBBARD, Sanjay Manohar, and Vilayanur Ramachandran developed a test to find out what really triggers grapheme-color synesthesia. Subjects concentrated on an ambiguous written character that looked somewhere between a "5" and an "S." When the character appeared in a string of chronological numbers, synesthetes saw the color of 5; when it appeared in a string of alphabetical letters, they saw the color of S. "It's not the visual properties of five that makes you see the color," Simner says. "It's the kind of five-ness of five, or the concept of five."

A more expansive, contemporary definition paints synesthesia as a merging of information that is otherwise unrelated and comes to a synesthete automatically; these aren't memorized connections, rather they're detailed, intense, and lifelong experiences. Synesthesia isn't something you can train your brain to have.

Another reason a purely sensory-based definition of synesthesia doesn't quite work is that cultural information can play an important role in how some kinds of synesthesia manifests, and that certainly goes beyond sensation. "You should know there's a ton of controversy around this," Simner says. "There are some scientists who are purists and they really want synesthesia to be sensory." Grapheme-personification synesthesia occurs when an individual understands numbers and letters as having consistent and detailed personalities. While the general personality types show up throughout historical documentation of synesthesia—a shy number or a bossy letter—the cultural references that people use to describe their graphemes change with the times.

"There are records of people with personification synesthesia going back into the 19th century who reported their letters and numbers were society girls and suffragettes," Simner says. "Today, personified graphemes are Instagrammers, YouTubers, or club bouncers."

Synesthesia is a merging of information that is otherwise unrelated and comes to a synesthete automatically; these aren't memorized connections . . . synesthesia isn't something you can train your brain to have.

Synesthesia allows Lucy Cordes Engelman to see time as colored geometric shapes. Daniel Mullen's art represents her aerial view of a century changing; zero is white.

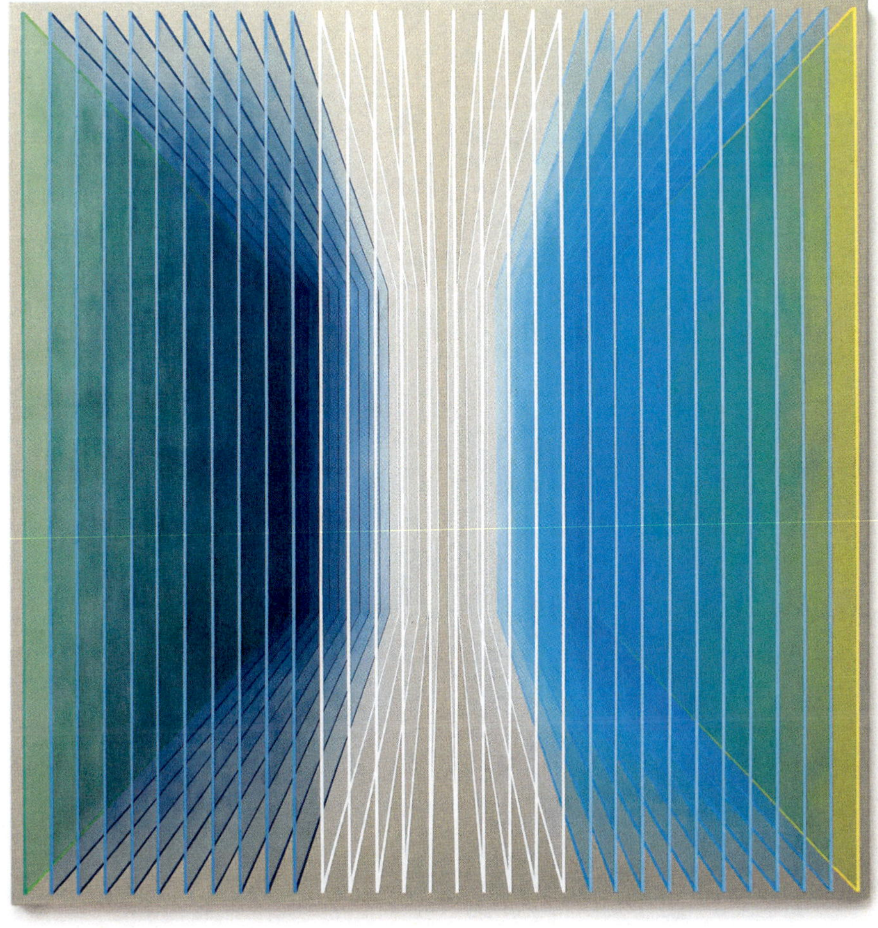

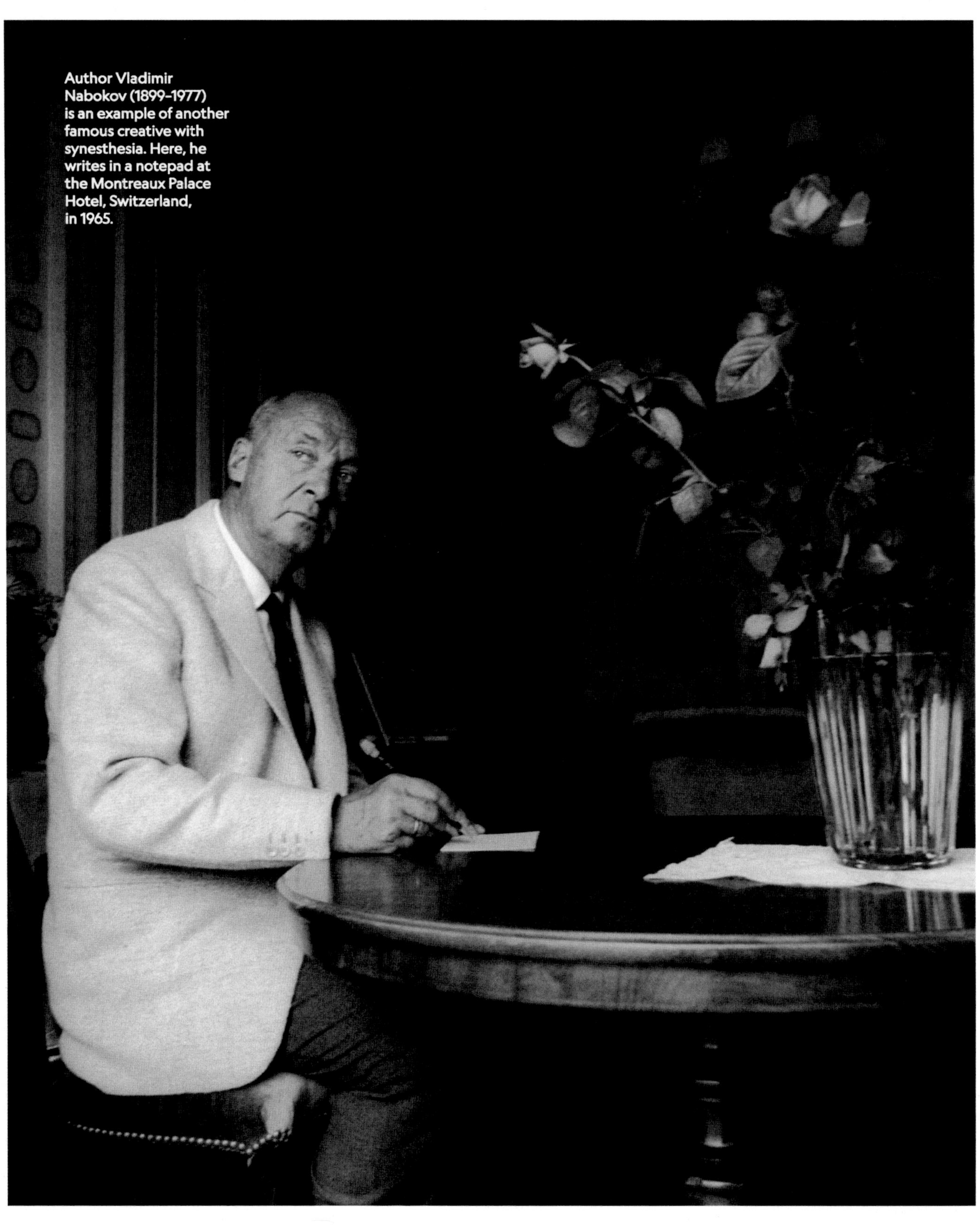
Author Vladimir Nabokov (1899–1977) is an example of another famous creative with synesthesia. Here, he writes in a notepad at the Montreaux Palace Hotel, Switzerland, in 1965.

POINTY CHICKEN AND fMRIs

ALTHOUGH SYNESTHESIA HAD been documented for hundreds of years, it wasn't until the 1990s that the scientific research supporting its existence really began to take off. The tipping point was the confluence of an influential researcher and a surge in technological advancements. In 1980, the neurologist Richard Cytowic had a now-famous dinner with a friend who declared, "Oh, dear, there aren't enough points on the chicken." That comment by a synesthete who tasted shapes launched Cytowic's curiosity, and his influential research in turn shot synesthesia into the zeitgeist.

By the early 2000s, researchers across many fields of neuroscience began using functional magnetic resonance imaging, or fMRI, which scans and maps activity in discrete regions of the brain. For synesthesia researchers, the tool showed consistent differences between the brains of synesthetes and nonsynesthetes in both brain activity and structure. When grapheme-color synesthetes look at monochrome numbers while within an fMRI machine, scientists can see the color-selective region of their visual cortices activate. And when people with grapheme-personification synesthesia look at monochrome numbers, their brains' corpus callosum, which aids in social processing, activates. Synesthetes also have higher white matter connectivity—increased wiring in their brains (the same tracts that are dampened in prosopagnosics). In all cases, the brains of control subjects without synesthesia showed none of these features.

Most studies rely on synesthetes who come forward knowing their diagnosis already, which can lead to lowball estimates of how many synesthetes there are in the world. Proactively screening for synesthesia is a better method. Simner has screened 20,000 people in her career. In the 1990s, the prevalence was estimated at one in 2,000 people—today, the estimate is around one in 25. Within the global population, that would mean there are about 312 million synesthetes worldwide (the population of the United States, for comparison, is 332 million people).

Yet the origin of this transfixing ability remains highly debated. In the

THE BRAIN'S RELAY STATION

Nestled at the center of the brain is the thalamus. Its robust nerve connections to the cerebral cortex and the midbrain make it like air traffic control: Sensations about the world around you are processed here, then sent on to whatever area of the brain can best deal with each one. The thalamus's unique wiring enables it to sift through higher-order cortical functions, such as decision-making, and subcortical functions such as emotions. If you walk up to a ledge, estimate the drop, feel scared, and step back, the thalamus is coordinating the whole experience. This central hub may also be critical in causing synesthesia. Some scientists hypothesize that synesthesia arises partly from robust connections in the thalamus sustained during development, leaving the brain able to weave experiences. Synesthetes are born this way, but in a few rare cases, a person who sustained a thalamic injury acquired synesthesia.

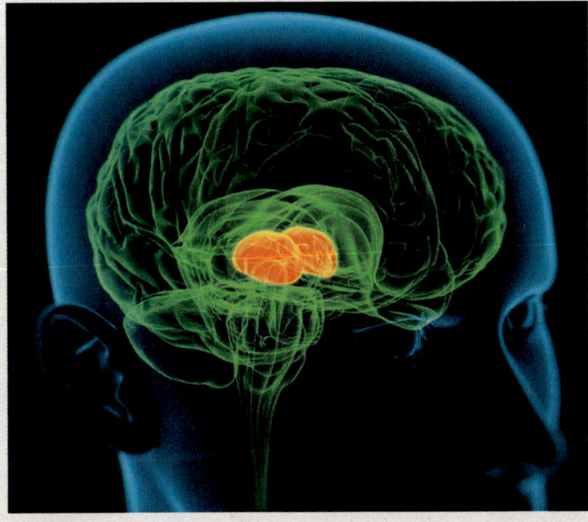

The thalamus—shown in red, atop the brainstem—is an important relay station for sensation and motor signals.

early 1990s, Daphne Maurer, a developmental psychologist, hypothesized that all newborns experience synesthesia. Humans are born with hyperconnected brains that become less so with development and age—a healthy process called pruning, during which unnecessary neuronal connections snap with disuse. Maurer concluded that in some people this hyperconnectivity remains, giving rise to lifelong synesthesia beyond infancy.

THE MAIN HANG-UP about this hypothesis is that the theory has never been tested and probably never will be because there's no way to identify synesthetes from birth—and even if you could identify them, someone would have to then test and track those people for life. Not having that data is too much of a leap for some scientists.

Despite this, Simner, the neuropsychologist, is moving the needle a bit by spearheading the first longitudinal study of children with synesthesia. While it still doesn't answer the question of where synesthesia comes from, tracking a child through time offers a better understanding of how synesthesia impacts development, as well as how to better diagnose and support those with this ability. "I do know of many, many cases where children are disbelieved, or where teachers have ridiculed them," Simner says.

In her longitudinal study—which includes papers published in 2006 and 2013—Simner has followed 615 children between the ages of six and 10 who are grapheme-color synesthetes. Over five years, she found that synesthetic children tend to be more anxious and more sensitive to light and noise than other children.

"So that's the bad news," Simner says. "But the rest is good news." They have better vocabulary skills—both in understanding and producing words—better memory spans, a heightened ability to reconstruct spatial patterns, and better "number guts," or the ability to quickly determine the quantity of something without counting. Other studies that have tracked adults with synesthesia found these perceptions do seem to dim with age, almost the way individual senses do in general. An aging grapheme-color synesthete will see their mental colors become less luminous. But it never goes away. It's there, coloring a person's world for life.

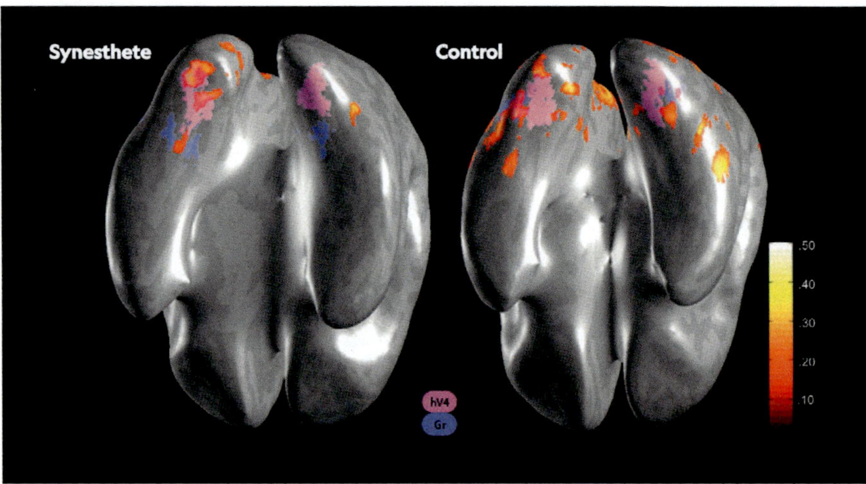

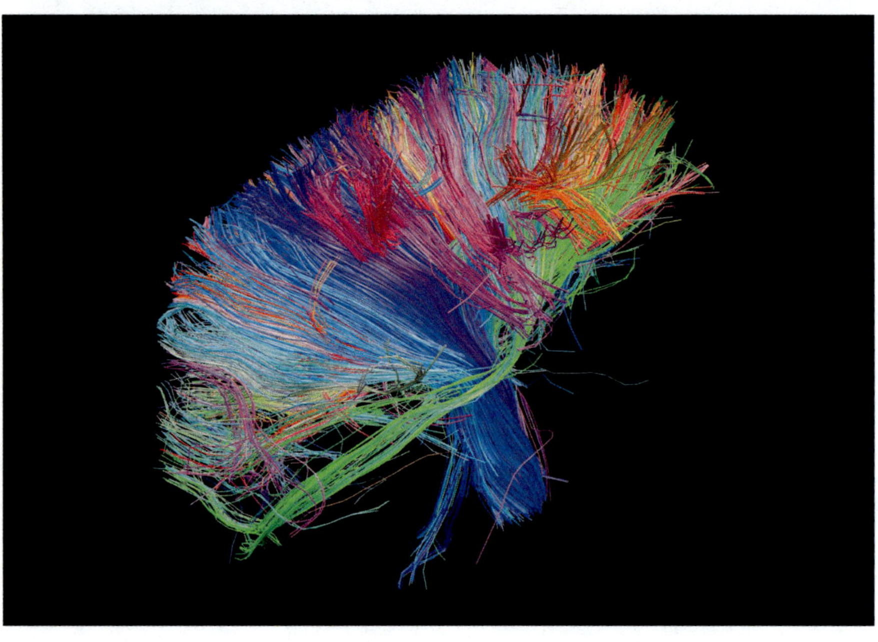

Top left: Some synesthetes perceive color when shown monochrome symbols. Color-sensing brain regions are marked purple in this landmark 2005 fMRI image. *Bottom left:* Synesthetes have denser white matter than the typical brain as shown in this image from the USC Stevens Neuroimaging and Informatics Institute for the Human Connectome Project.

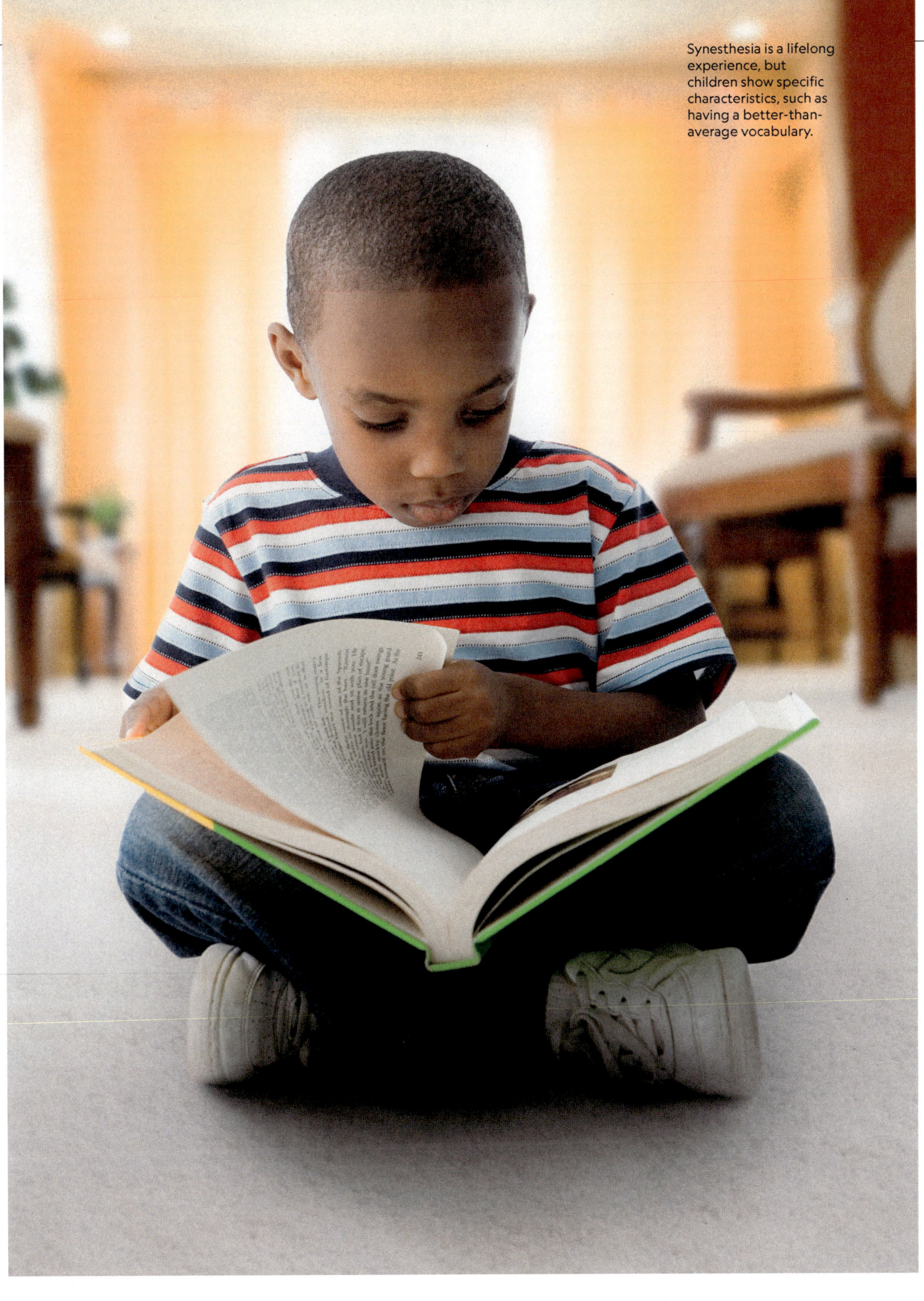

Synesthesia is a lifelong experience, but children show specific characteristics, such as having a better-than-average vocabulary.

CHAPTER 2

THE FLAVOR ILLUSION

Food can be so much more than just salty, sweet, bitter, sour, and umami. It comes down to a series of tricks your brain plays on you.

Bite down on a perfectly ripe strawberry and the pure sweetness of the juice hits you first. Then comes something far more complex: Your tongue feels rough seeds punctuating soft fruit, and a hint of sour breaks through the sweetness. If you had to name it, the word "tang" may drift forward. This isn't exactly a taste, but some intangible quality that makes a strawberry go so well with whipped cream and hold its own as a bastion of summer. The strawberry-ness of a strawberry is hard to put into words, but somehow, even with your eyes closed, you know it instantly apart from a raspberry or a blueberry based on a swirl of perceptions that together form the complex and poignant experience of flavor. That this experience happens immediately is a finely tuned dance of the senses that would be impossible without the brain as its choreographer.

The only thing scientists who study flavor agree on is what flavor is not. It's not a standalone sense like taste. But a unifying definition of what flavor is continues to escape those who study it. The purists among them think this multisensory experience arises simply from the brain combining the sensations of smell and taste. The progressives of the group regard flavor as bringing together smell, taste, and mouthfeel—the physical quality of food as the tongue touches it. And the scientific experimentalists see flavor as something even bigger.

Flavor is a complex illusion, beyond simple taste, and the brain pulls all the strings. The strawberry-ness of a strawberry comes from a combination of its texture, smell, taste, and possibly even color, depending who you ask. This important system is deeply tied to nutrition and survival.

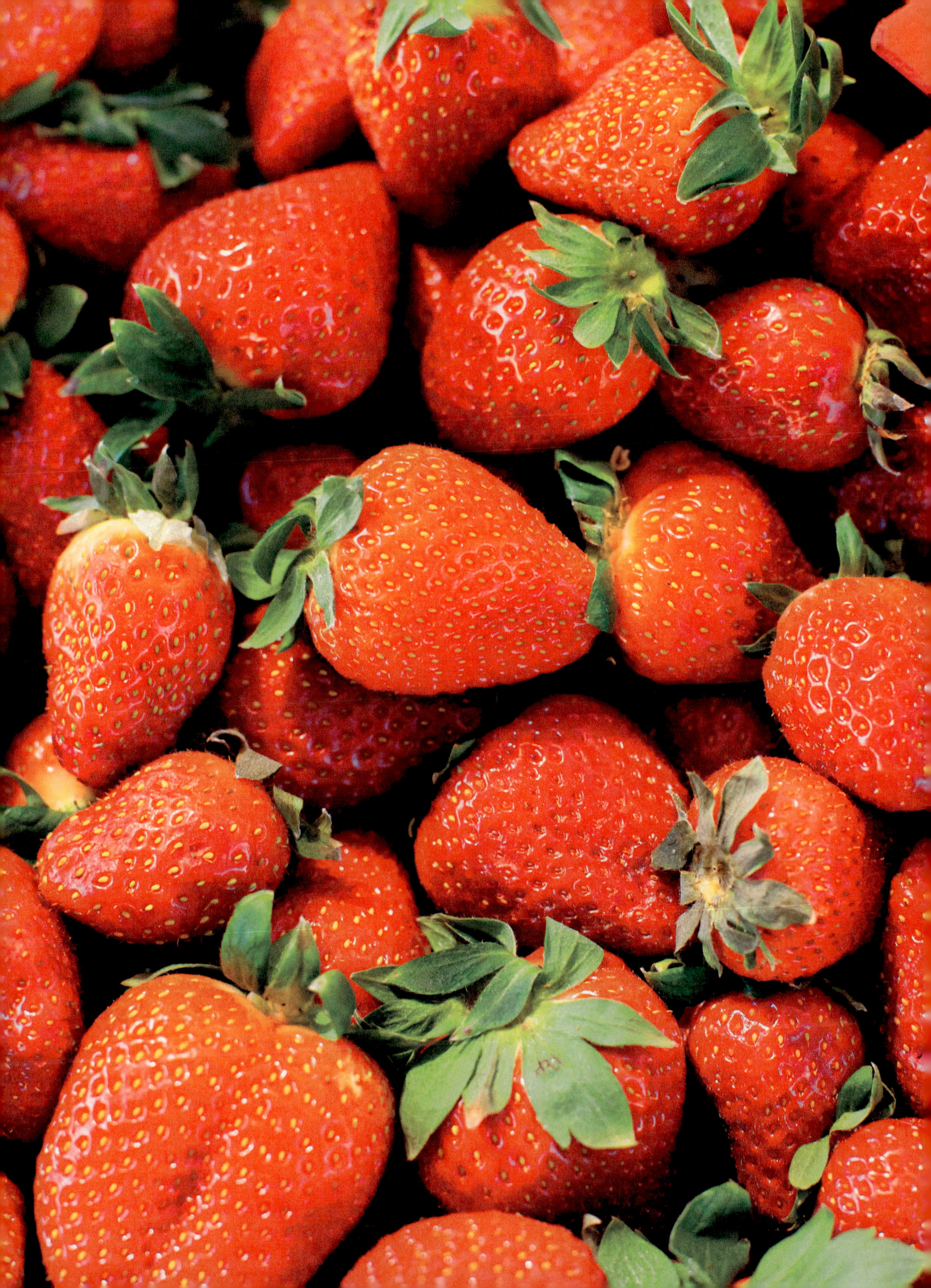

it's very interesting that we do not have an agreed-upon definition," says Small.

Then there's Gordon Shepherd's view on the debate. He made a monumental discovery about smell in the early 2000s that changed neuroscience and paved the way for a hybrid discipline called neurogastronomy. "Flavor is created by the brain," he says simply and with awe still.

Although it's hard to imagine, there is no flavor intrinsic to food, just as objects do not contain color but rather reflect wavelengths of light that we interpret as yellow, red, blue, and so on. It's our big, complex, interconnected brain that makes flavor—this delightful, disgusting, memorable, and emotional experience—and links it to food. Without the brain, a peak season strawberry would be nothing special at all.

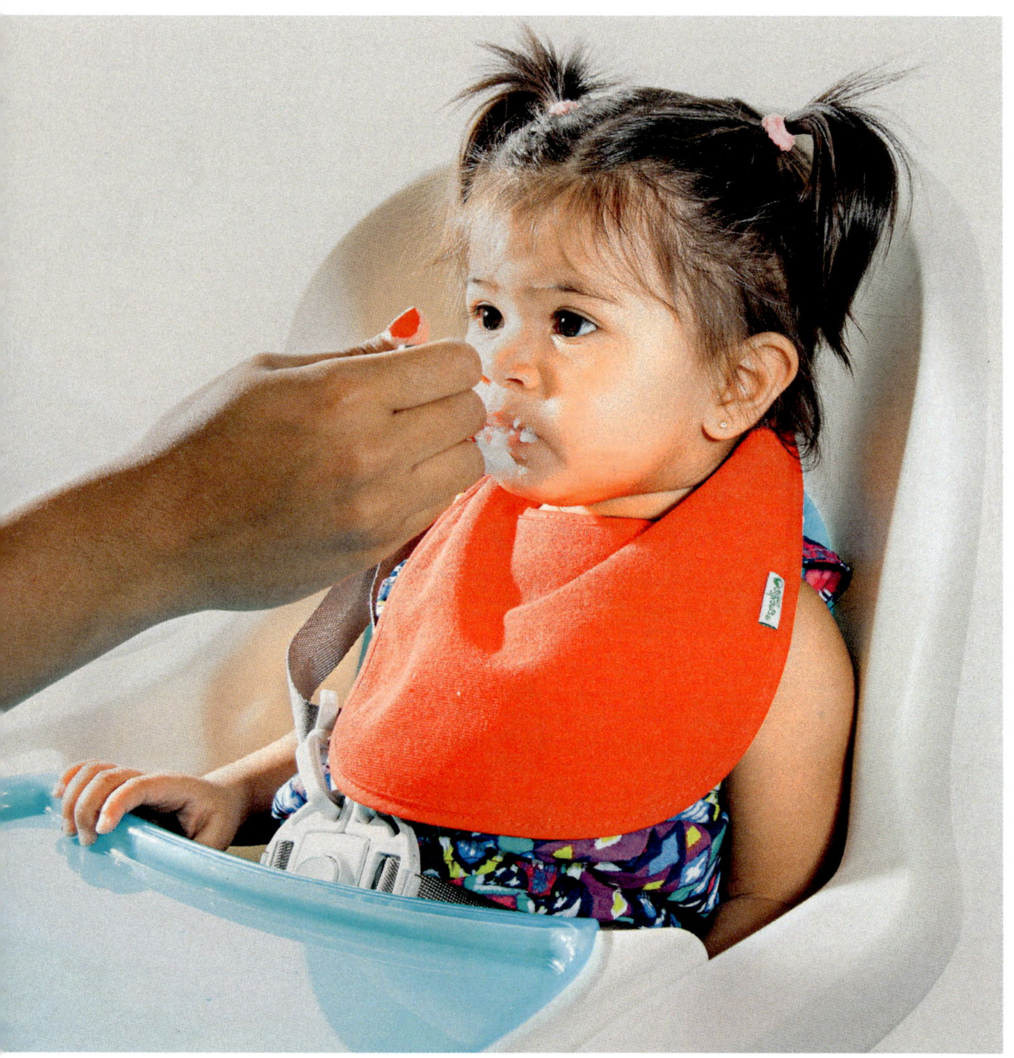

At the Monell Chemical Senses Center in Philadelphia, a baby girl has first-time food encounters. Although some of our flavor-experiencing system is intrinsic, it's also possible to expertly train the brain beyond that, as with sommeliers.

"I think flavor involves also vision and hearing," says Qian Janice Wang, assistant professor of food science at Denmark's Aarhus University. But, she concedes, "I'm sure that everyone you talk to might give you a different definition."

DANA SMALL, a neuroscientist at Yale University who studies how the brain mediates our behavior toward food, is open to the idea that the sound of eating a food—the auditory experience of a crunch, for example, not just the textural sensation of it—may directly play into flavor perception. But she rejects including the role of vision as integral to flavor. Seeing a steak dyed green would surely change your behavior toward eating it, but that's separate from the sensory experience that happens once you do eat the food. "I think

TASTE VERSUS FLAVOR

TASTE AND FLAVOR aren't the same thing. Specialized receptors on the tongue give rise to the five sensations that comprise taste: salty, sour, bitter, sweet, and umami. Any experience of food more complex than that falls into the realm of flavor. This is crucial, yet the way most people talk about what they eat or drink lags behind the physiological reality.

"When people say something tastes good, they usually mean its flavor is good or its sensory properties are good," says Robin Dando, associate professor of food science at Cornell

University, where he studies how humans evaluate food using their senses. But a few minutes later, even he—an expert—starts slipping up in the middle of a conversation about defining these very terms; it's a hard colloquialism to break. "I'm saying taste, and I'm dropping back into this language that I tell my students not to use," he says laughing.

Beyond confusing taste and flavor, language hides another mix-up, this time between taste and smell. The bulk of flavor actually comes from hundreds of receptors in the layer of skin that lines the nose—the olfactory epithelium—not the tongue. When someone says something tastes aromatic, what they really mean is it smells that way, yet the sensation seems to be coming from the mouth, says Jessleen Kanwal, a postdoctoral fellow at Caltech. It's perplexing, to say the least, but here's how this mix-up begins.

Chewing a tasty morsel with your teeth releases volatile compounds, chemical signatures of food that evaporate up into the back of the nasal cavity where nose and mouth join. As you eat, you exhale out through your nose, which pulls these compounds along a current of air from the mouth directly onto receptors in the nose's olfactory epithelium; such receptors can detect

Taste starts with receptors on the tongue called taste buds, shown here as pale dots in a sea of blue dye. Chewing food releases chemicals that bind with these receptors, sending information to the brain about whether the food is salty, sweet, sour, bitter, or umami.

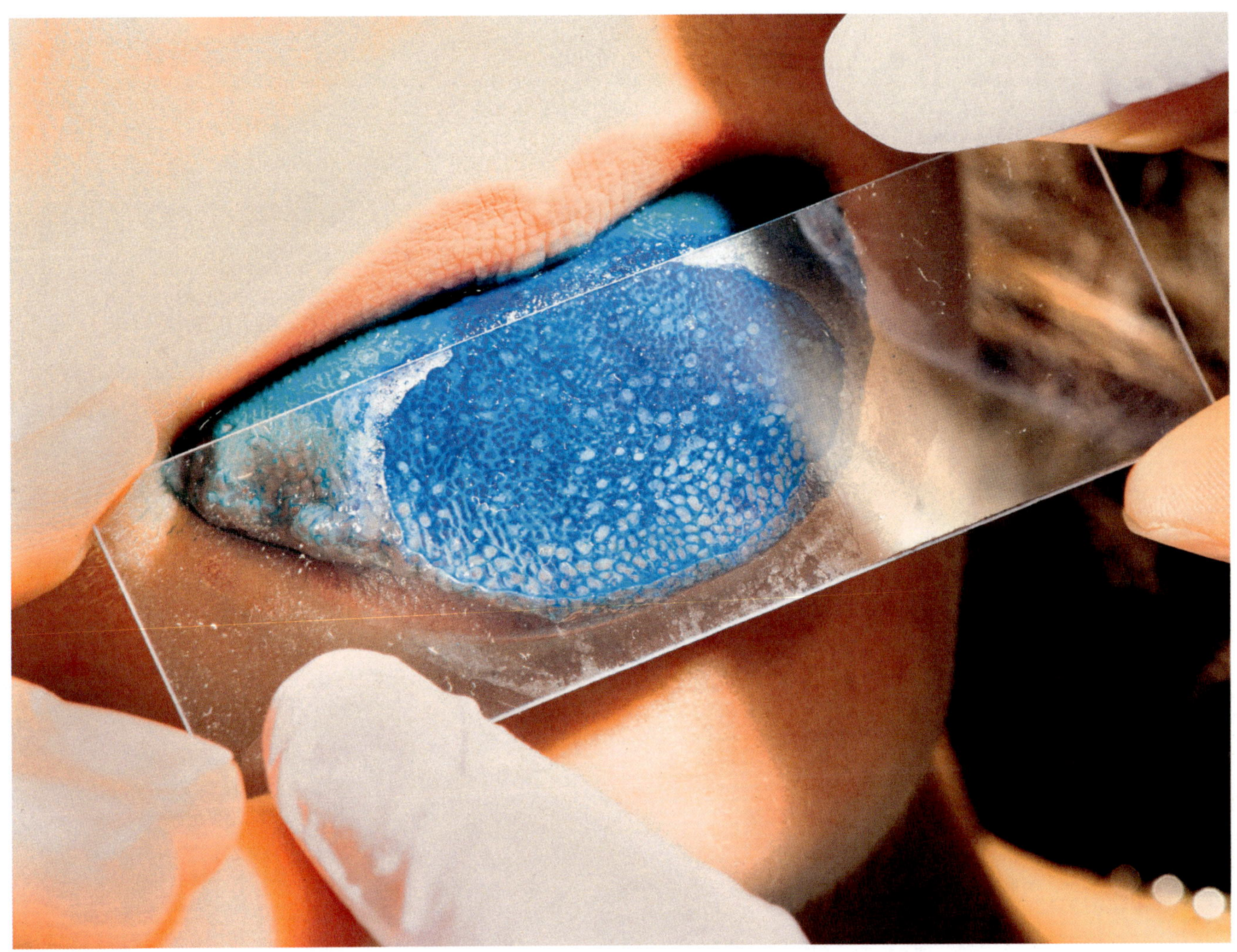

More Than Taste

HOW THE BRAIN CONSTRUCTS FLAVOR

The tongue detects basic tastes, but the nose—with hundreds of receptors for chemicals that waft off food—contributes more to flavor. According to neurobiologist Gordon Shepherd, the brain draws on all the senses to assemble a complex "flavor image" that lingers in our memory.

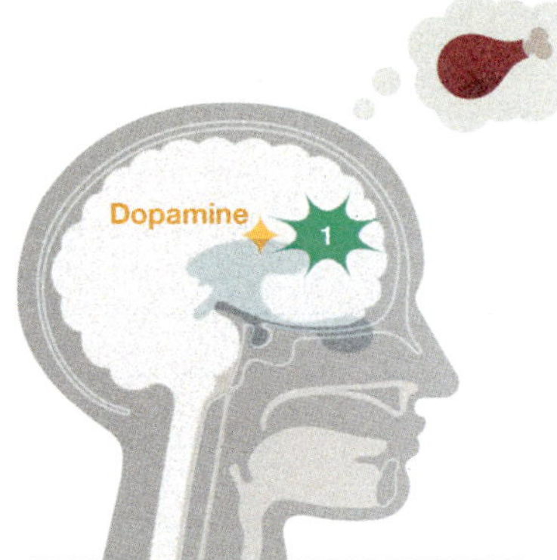

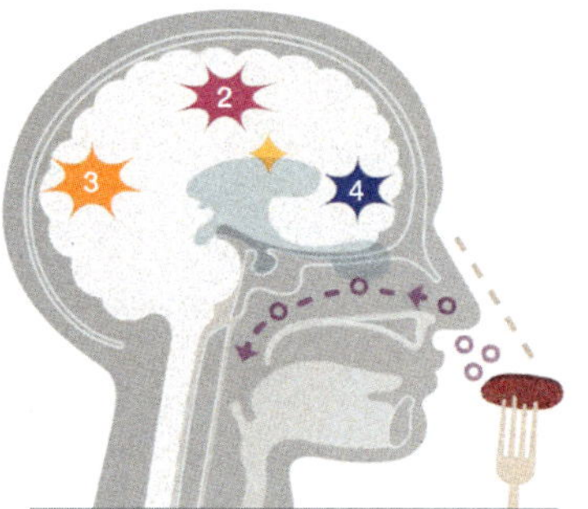

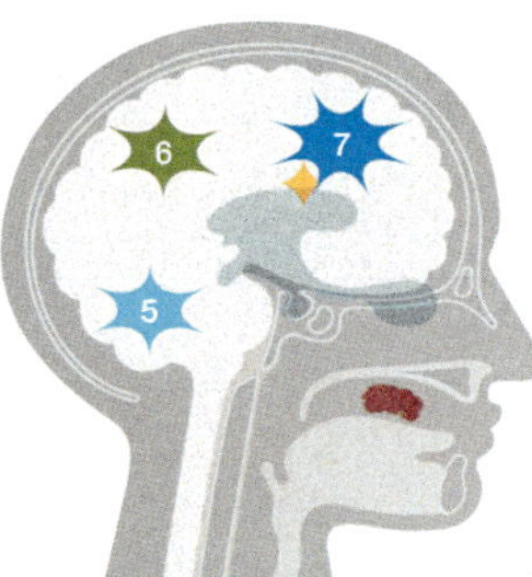

ANTICIPATION

A flavor experience may begin with a past meal: The memory 1 activates dopamine reward centers, leading us to crave the flavors to come. We salivate.

SENSORY OVERTURE

A brain primed for pleasure begins to receive sensory impulses from the food as we move it to our mouth 2, see its colors and shapes 3, and inhale its aroma 4.

SOUNDS DELICIOUS

We chew. Sound 5 and mouthfeel 6 add key information: Is the food gooey, crunchy, or crispy? Receptors in our taste buds register sweet, salty, sour, bitter, and umami 7.

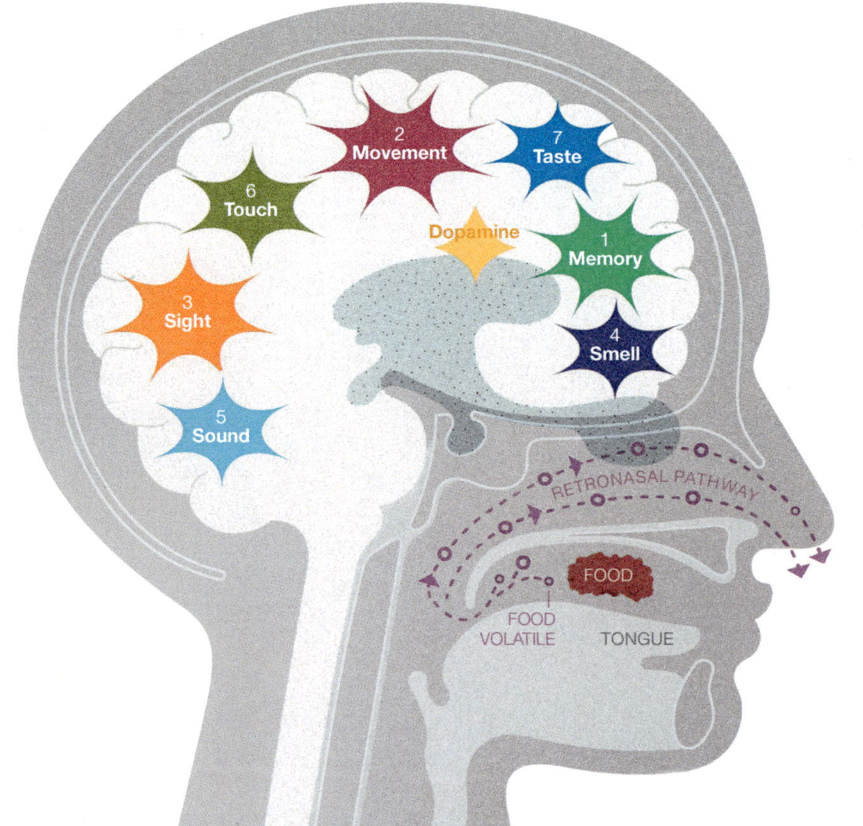

SENSATIONS MERGE TO CREATE FLAVOR

Volatile chemicals waft off food as we chew and swallow it, and as we exhale, they're carried into the nasal cavity from behind. The brain combines information from all the senses to produce the experience of flavor. And though we think it originates in the mouth, most of it actually comes from these "retronasal" smells detected by receptors in the nose. They build the memory that prepares us for the next experience.

JOHN TOMANIO, NGM STAFF; SHELLEY SPERRY
ART: SCRIPT & SEAL
SOURCE: GORDON SHEPHERD, YALE UNIVERSITY

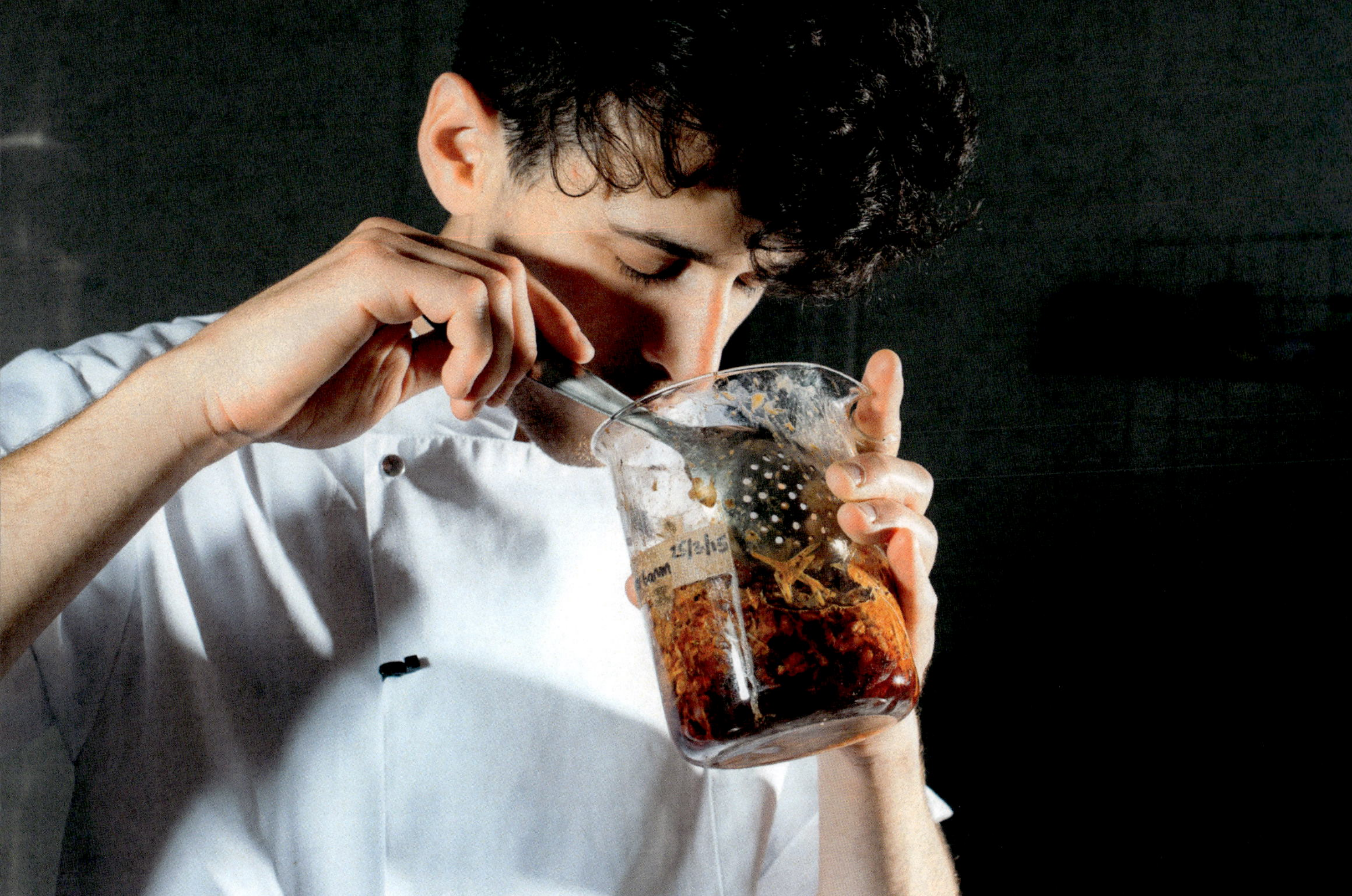

A food scientist inhales strained fermented insect garum at a food lab in Denmark. Smell is key to flavor, but the brain tricks us into thinking flavor comes from the mouth.

thousands of meaningfully distinct odorants. This covert process, called retronasal smell, works the opposite way from the smelling we tend to think of ourselves as doing. That's orthonasal smell, in which we sniff inward to detect odorants in our environment.

The concept of retronasal smell upended conventional thinking in 2006, when Shepherd first published a paper on how it works in the journal *Nature*. Compared to the tongue, which can sense only five tastes, the nose is a far more crucial tool in having a complex relationship with food. You can test this on yourself by closing your eyes, holding your nose, and consuming a slice of apple, and then a slice of potato. Suddenly, these two wildly different types of produce become indistinguishable.

A NOSE FOR FLAVOR

THE COMPLEXITY OF smell has enabled hundreds of distinct global cuisines to emerge, a feat that would be impossible if we had only taste at our disposal. The nose is the first biological step in making Kansas City BBQ sauce completely, identifiably different from Texas BBQ sauce—and even that's a simplification, as within these communities there are variations still. Yet the nose's role in all this delicious complexity languishes in obscurity.

"We derive so much knowledge from vision and hearing that I feel like there is a lack of appreciation for how much knowledge we can derive from smell,"

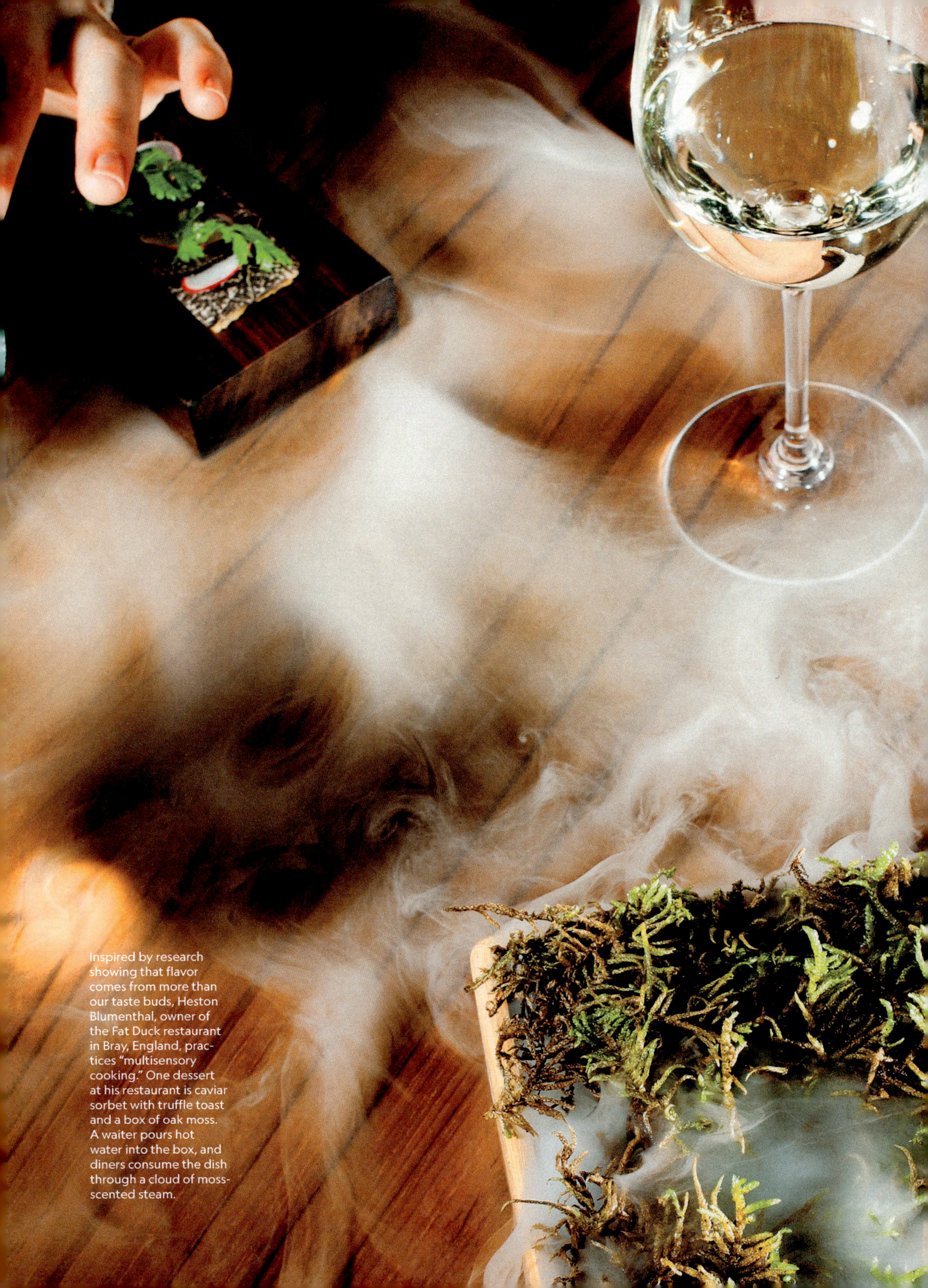

Inspired by research showing that flavor comes from more than our taste buds, Heston Blumenthal, owner of the Fat Duck restaurant in Bray, England, practices "multisensory cooking." One dessert at his restaurant is caviar sorbet with truffle toast and a box of oak moss. A waiter pours hot water into the box, and diners consume the dish through a cloud of moss-scented steam.

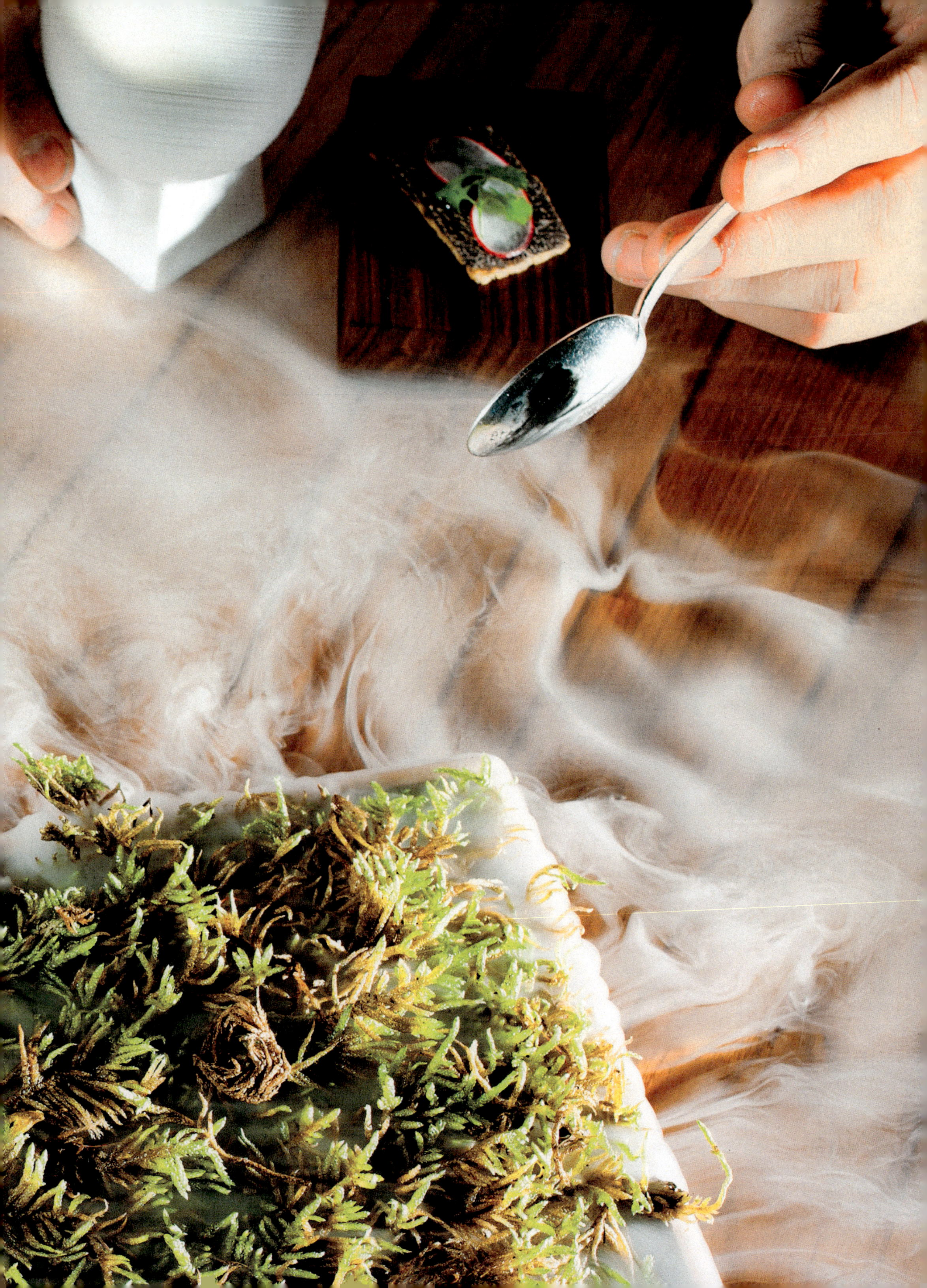

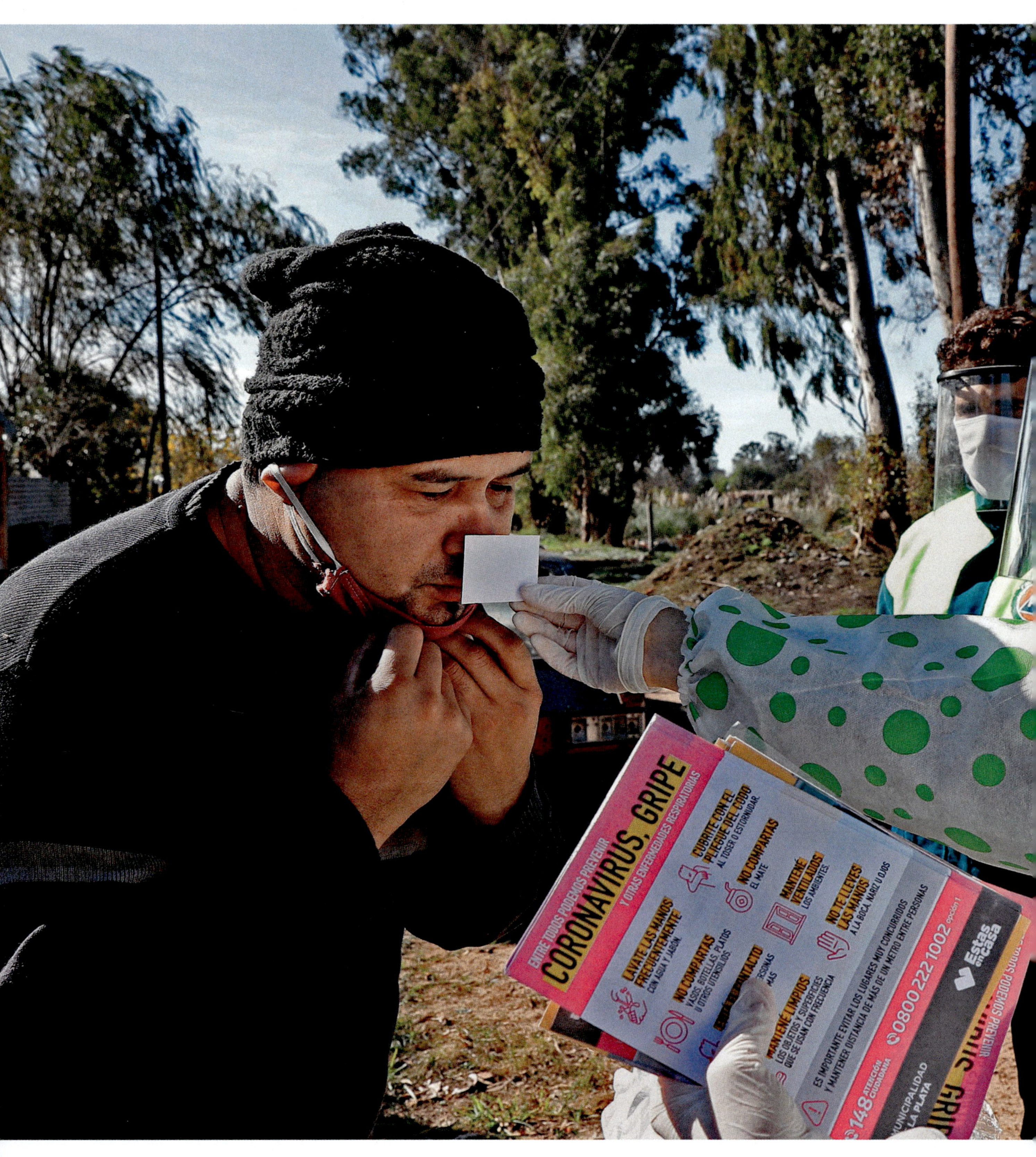
ENTRE TODOS PODEMOS PREVENIR
CORONAVIRUS, GRIPE
Y OTRAS ENFERMEDADES RESPIRATORIAS
LAVATE LAS MANOS FRECUENTEMENTE
CON AGUA Y JABÓN
CUBRITE CON EL PLIEGUE DEL CODO
AL TOSER O ESTORNUDAR.
NO COMPARTAS
VASOS, BOTELLAS, PLATOS U OTROS UTENSILIOS
NO COMPARTAS
EL MATE
MANTENÉ VENTILADOS
LOS AMBIENTES.
NO TE LLEVES LAS MANOS
A LA BOCA, NARIZ U OJOS
MANTENÉ LIMPIOS
LOS OBJETOS Y SUPERFICIES QUE SE USAN CON FRECUENCIA
ES IMPORTANTE EVITAR LOS LUGARES MUY CONCURRIDOS
Y MANTENER DISTANCIA DE MÁS DE UN METRO ENTRE PERSONAS
148 ATENCIÓN CIUDADANA
0800 222 1002 opción 1
Estas en casa
LA PLATA

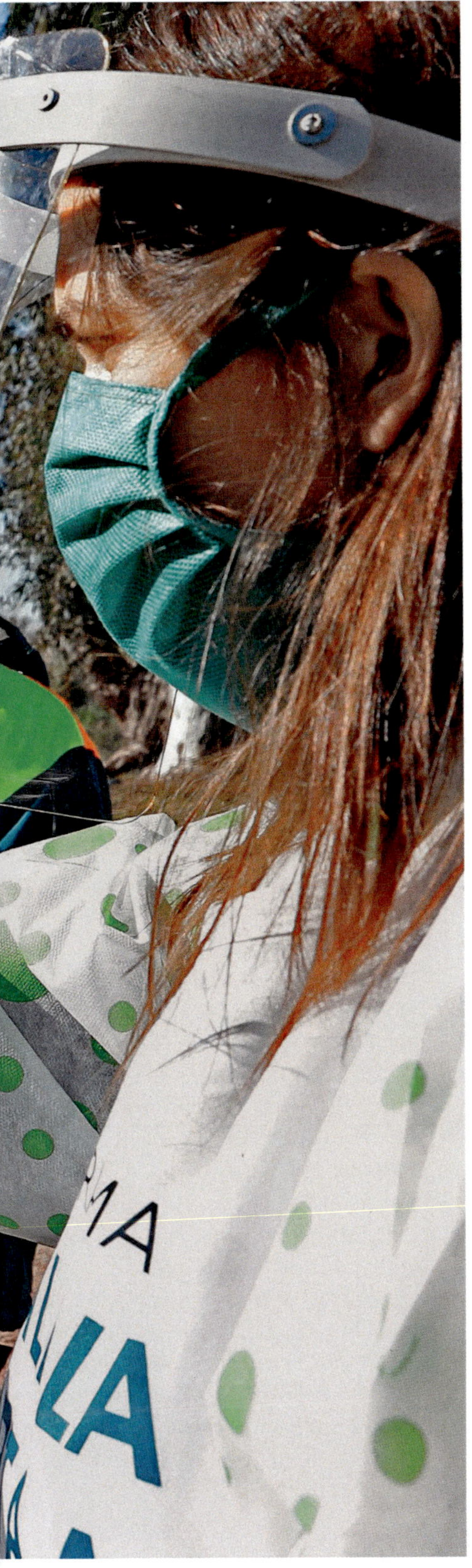

Health care workers near Buenos Aires, Argentina, used smell tests to track COVID-19 in May 2020. Loss of smell—and thus flavor—is a symptom of infection.

says Wang, the experimental food scientist. "Not just, 'Oh, this is rotten,' or, 'What does it smell like?' but really quite sophisticated knowledge."

We humans tend to think of ourselves as subpar smellers, especially compared to dogs, and assume smell doesn't play a heavy role in how we experience life. But as the COVID-19 pandemic has shown, a negative health experience can quickly put things back into perspective. Thousands have lost their ability to enjoy food because of the way the novel coronavirus attacks the sensitive smell system. Major health agencies, such as the CDC, list a common symptom of COVID-19 infection as "loss of taste and smell."

In reality, loss of taste is an incredibly rare experience, and what's most often lost is solely the sense of smell, and with it, flavor. Despite the colloquial phrasing of the symptoms, the immense scale of the pandemic has pushed to the forefront just how important fully perceiving food is. As a secondary outcome of a disease, or treatment, loss of smell has historically been put on the back burner while physicians handle the primary disease. But it's increasingly gaining traction as a major quality of life issue, as well as a covert symptom that could be highly useful in catching oncoming disease early.

"It turns out that the olfactory system in the brain is sort of like a canary in the mineshaft," says Shepherd. Colds and sinus infections can block the flow of air critical for the retronasal smell that gives rise to flavor. Loss of smell is also a common side effect in chemotherapy, an imprecise treatment used most often to target rapidly dividing cancer cells. Other cells in the body that also regenerate quickly, such as olfactory neurons, are civilian casualties in chemo's toxic blitz. Increasing bodies of research also point to loss of smell—often noticed when someone loses their appetite—as an important early sign of Alzheimer's disease and Parkinson's.

"If we want to understand how to potentially improve their conditions, it's really important that we know how the brain is organized and actually processes all of that information to begin with," says Kanwal, the Caltech postdoc. Complex thought and decision-making take place in the brain's orbitofrontal cortex after information passes through several lower-order neural areas first, and scientists often point to this region as the formative flavor center. This model assumes the brain is processing each sense individually before combining them to create flavor. But in Kanwal's previous research, when she was getting her PhD at Harvard University, she found that fruit fly brains actually integrate smell and taste into one "flavor" impulse almost

Compared to the tongue, which can sense only five tastes, the nose is a far more crucial tool in having a complex relationship with food.

immediately. It may seem odd to look to a minuscule insect for clues about the human brain, but the fruit fly's olfactory system is quite similar to that of mammals. "That really changes the way we think about how the brain is organized," says Kanwal.

When people who lose their ability to perceive flavor describe the experience of eating, they often compare it to living in black and white. Even with imprecise language that confuses taste and flavor, and taste and smell, when we lose the ability to smell, there is still an emotional understanding that, with only taste, food becomes flat and uninviting. But one reason this is rarely articulated may be because the brain is tricking us into perceiving retronasal smell, and thus flavor, as coming entirely from the mouth.

THE IMPORTANCE OF ILLUSIONS

HOW YOU COGNITIVELY perceive the world is actually a pretty poor representation of the way the world is in reality. The kind of gimmicky optical illusions featured in children's science books—such as staring at a static picture of a circular checkerboard and perceiving the rows as spinning in alternate directions—are the best known of these perceptual mistellings, but we all encounter them throughout the day in other sensory systems and in such highly assimilated ways that we're likely unaware they're even happening.

Watching television activates such a spell. You experience the sound of the actors speaking as coming directly from their mouths, but if you stop to think about what you know of how a television works, that doesn't make sense. The sound, of course, is coming out of the television speakers,

TIME TRAVEL ON A WHIFF

Taste, touch, sight, hearing, and smell all begin as a response to an event occurring outside the body, whether that's seeing a flash of lightning or hearing a song. The first four sensations pass through the brain's relay station, the thalamus, before encountering emotion and memory processing in the amygdala and hippocampus, and then moving on to the cortex, where senses start to become complex experiences. That's how you might come to fear lightning rather than merely see it. Smell is the only sense that gets to bypass this system.

Olfactory neurons that detect smells in the environment have a direct line to emotion and memory. Research shows that the brain forms the strongest smell-linked memories before the age of 10, so the smell of sharpened pencils would more likely take you back to a moment in a kindergarten art class than to an exam in high school. This special anatomy is also why the briefest whiff of that pencil transports you back in a way that seeing the sharpened pencil won't.

Because chewing releases volatile compounds that are actually processed as smells, not tastes, food is an especially powerful tool for triggering these strong memories. One hypothesis for the unparalleled connectivity of our olfactory system is the evolutionary benefit of smell as a tool for sussing out danger as well as potential mates, both critical for species survival.

Smell is our oldest sense and has the receptor bulk to show for it: While human eyes have two types of receptors for sensing light and sending information to the brain, the human nose has about 400 types of receptors to pick up odors.

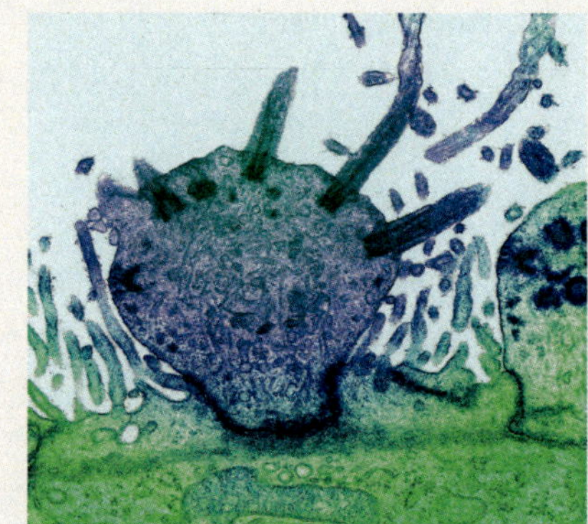

Nasal olfactory receptors send smell information to the brain.

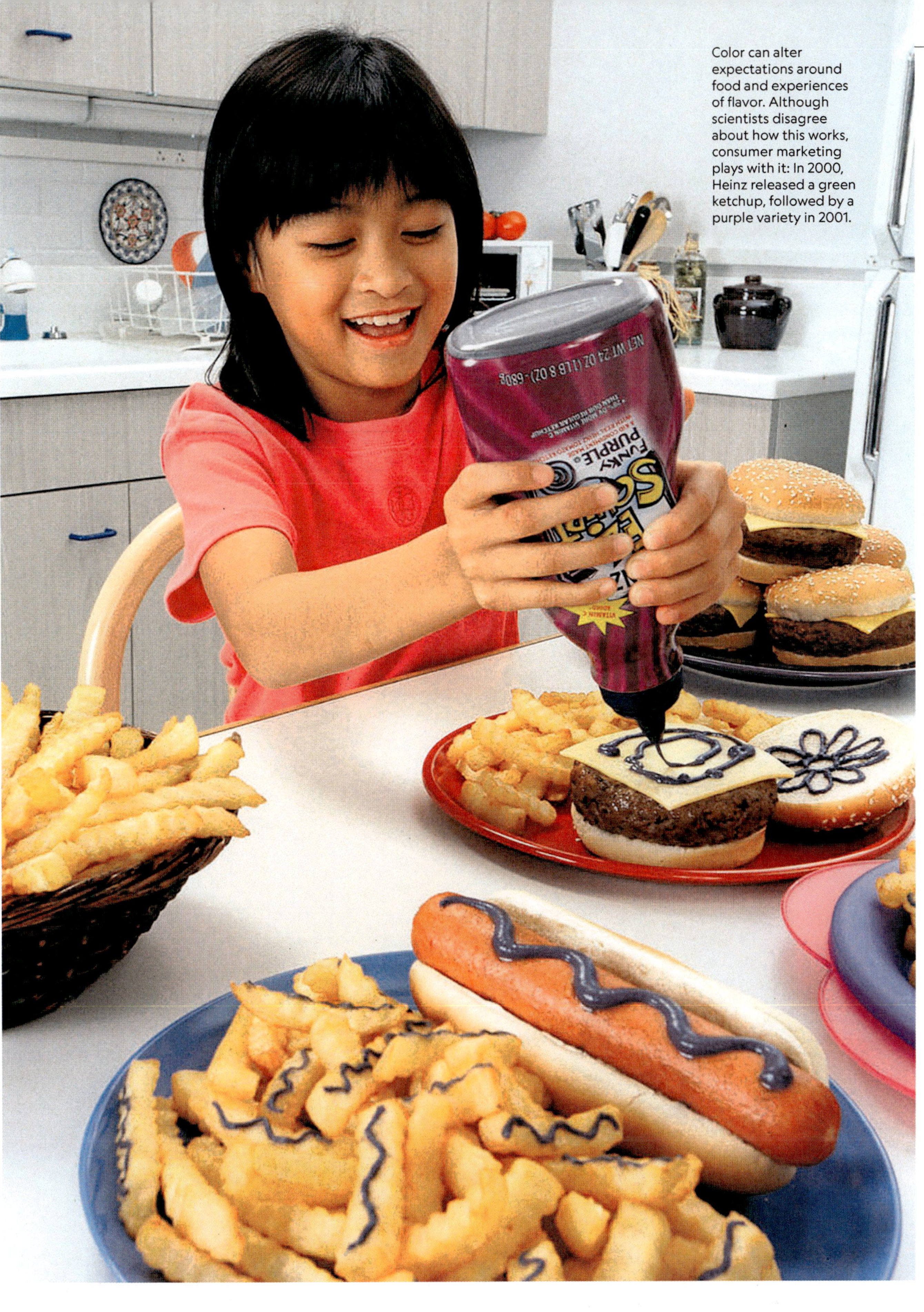

Color can alter expectations around food and experiences of flavor. Although scientists disagree about how this works, consumer marketing plays with it: In 2000, Heinz released a green ketchup, followed by a purple variety in 2001.

separate from the moving image of a person talking. Because the sound and image are coming from roughly the same place in space and time, your brain makes the world a kinder, simpler place and you experience the two sensory inputs as being one event. This experience typifies where sensation ends and perception begins, says Small, the Yale neuroscientist. Only a technical difficulty might ruin the illusion—anyone with a streaming service and a bad internet connection knows the vexation of hearing spoken words out of sync with a moving mouth.

It's possible to manipulate our sense of taste: Food dyed pink, for example, tastes sweeter, even if it contains the same amount of sugar as a blue food.

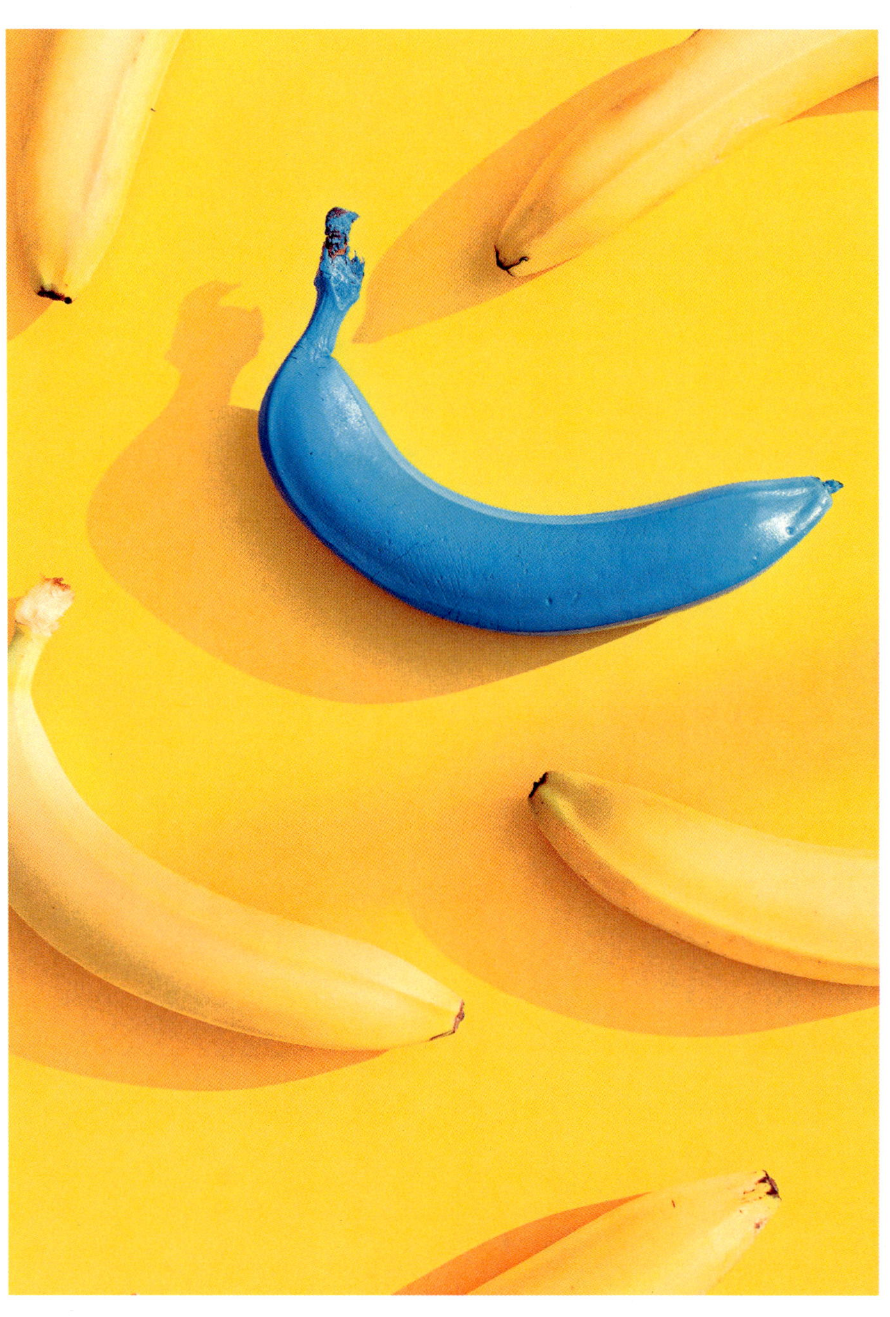

THE PERCEPTION THAT flavor is born in the mouth is another such daily illusion, a gastronomical trick the brain plays that belies how your body actually works. When you're chewing that ripe strawberry, receptors on the tongue relay chemical information about taste to the brain separately from receptors located in the nose, which are also relaying chemical information to the brain, but about smells. The brain receives both at about the same time, and from almost the same place on the body. The brain's somatomotor mouth area simplifies this process and tethers both sensations to the mouth. This experience is called the oral capture illusion. In doing this, the brain finely differentiates between information coming from the receptors at the back of the nose, those that sense chewing-related smells, and receptors at the front of the nose, those that sense smells in the environment. If the brain were to mix up the information from these two sets of receptors—which are physically only about one inch apart in your body—you'd perhaps experience the unpleasant smell of mothballs as though it were coming from your mouth.

"There are a lot of illusions that make up perception, and in this case the trickery makes a lot of sense," says Small. "It's basically imperfect physiology trying to do a better job at capturing reality." The reality is that as you eat, the strawberry you feel in

THE GUT-BRAIN AXIS

Clusters of nerve cells throughout your body run connections back and forth between the big brain in your skull and so-called little brains farther afield. The human digestive tract is the largest of these, home to 100 million nerve cells—called the enteric nervous system—paving a two-way communication highway to the brain's 86 billion nerve cells. While areas of the body dense with nerve cells can't generate complex cognition the way that similar groupings of cells in the brain can, they still have a lot of influence on mood and emotion.

Anxiety and depression are more common among people with irritable bowel syndrome (IBS) than in the general population, and scientists originally thought it was because this gut-brain axis went one way: that psychiatric mood disorders originating in the brain could choreograph malfunctions in the digestive tract, causing constipation, diarrhea, and abdominal pain. But new research flips this relationship, suggesting that disorders such as IBS can also cause anxiety and depression. Enteric nerve cells are primarily focused on helping you swallow and digest food when everything is working smoothly, but irritation in the gastrointestinal tract can nudge these cells to communicate with the central nervous system in a cascade that begets a sort of parallel irritation in the brain.

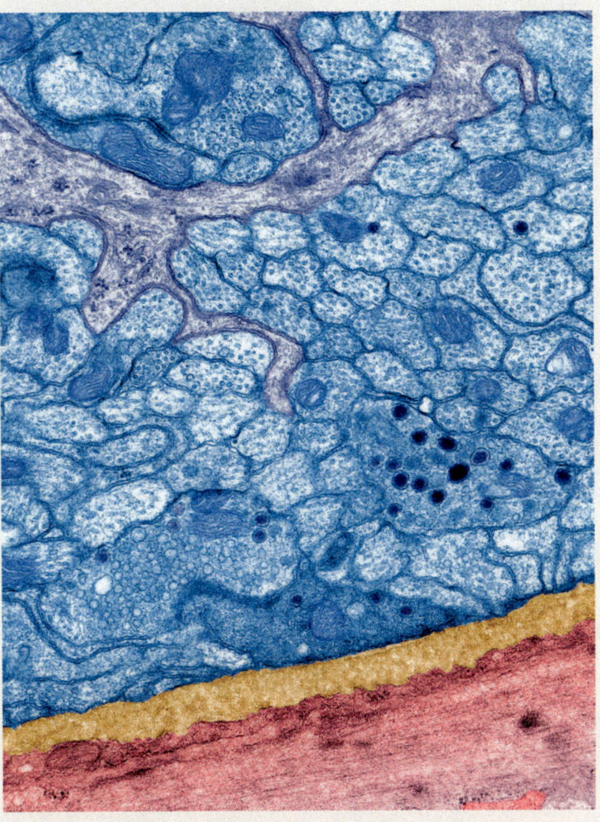

The enteric nervous system in the gut transmits information to the brain and vice versa.

Part of what makes IBS so tough to treat with dietary changes is how unpredictable the syndrome can be. Unlike celiac disease or food-specific allergies, IBS has no consistent trigger, such as gluten or peanuts. A person with IBS can have a perfectly fine meal one day and eat the exact same meal the next week only to find themselves holed up in the bathroom for hours afterward. With a better understanding of the gut-brain axis, more physicians are now prescribing low doses of tricyclic antidepressants to those with IBS, even if patients are not exhibiting any mood disorders. The medications act on nerve cells in the gut, blocking messages of pain they're trying to send to the brain. Disrupting this communication seems to calm symptoms of digestive distress in the process.

your mouth—and nowhere else on your body—does singularly contain all of these chemical compounds, even though the receptors for sensing them are in different places. "Imagine the evolution that has to happen in order to create oral capture illusions," says Small. "It's a lot of physiological gymnastics to go through, so it must have an important purpose."

The purpose, as she understands from both scientific and personal experience, is to help you differentiate nutrients from toxins in a highly sophisticated and nuanced way. "The classic example is conditioned taste aversion, which is actually conditioned *flavor* aversion," says Small.

When she was 19 years old—within the legal drinking age in her native Canada—Small celebrated the

A CLOSER LOOK

PLAYING WITH FOOD

One absurd and delicious dinner changed the course of food scientist Qian Janice Wang's life and research.

Something you should know about me is that I'm really into wine," says Qian Janice Wang emphatically. "Like, *really* into wine." Wang's life is full of flavor. A self-described foodie in her personal adventures, Wang also studies flavor perception in her professional life, as an assistant professor of food science at Aarhus University, a research institution on the east coast of Denmark's Jutland region.

One sip of wine holds vast amounts of chemical hints about its origins that pass right by the average drinker. Wang's attuned body, however, can translate it all into meaningful information: What was the climate like the year the grapes grew? What kind of vessels did the winemaker store the liquid in? Oak? Steel? And for how long? She's specially trained to crack this flavor code.

A Passion for Food

Wang originally set out to study music and emotion as a graduate student at the MIT Media Lab. "Food was a passion," she says, "but I didn't think that I could do research with food."

Then she and a group of friends road-tripped to Chicago's renowned restaurant, Alinea, which specializes in molecular gastronomy, a playful, scientific approach to food that pushes it to a place where the word "dinner" doesn't suffice anymore. Wang remembers a

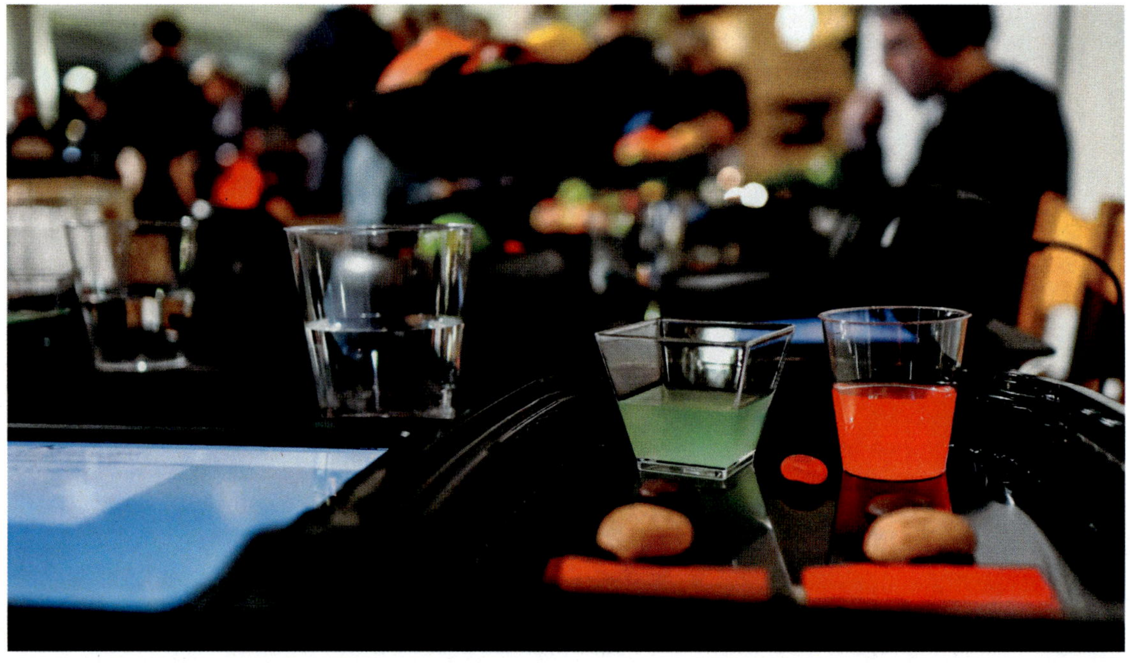

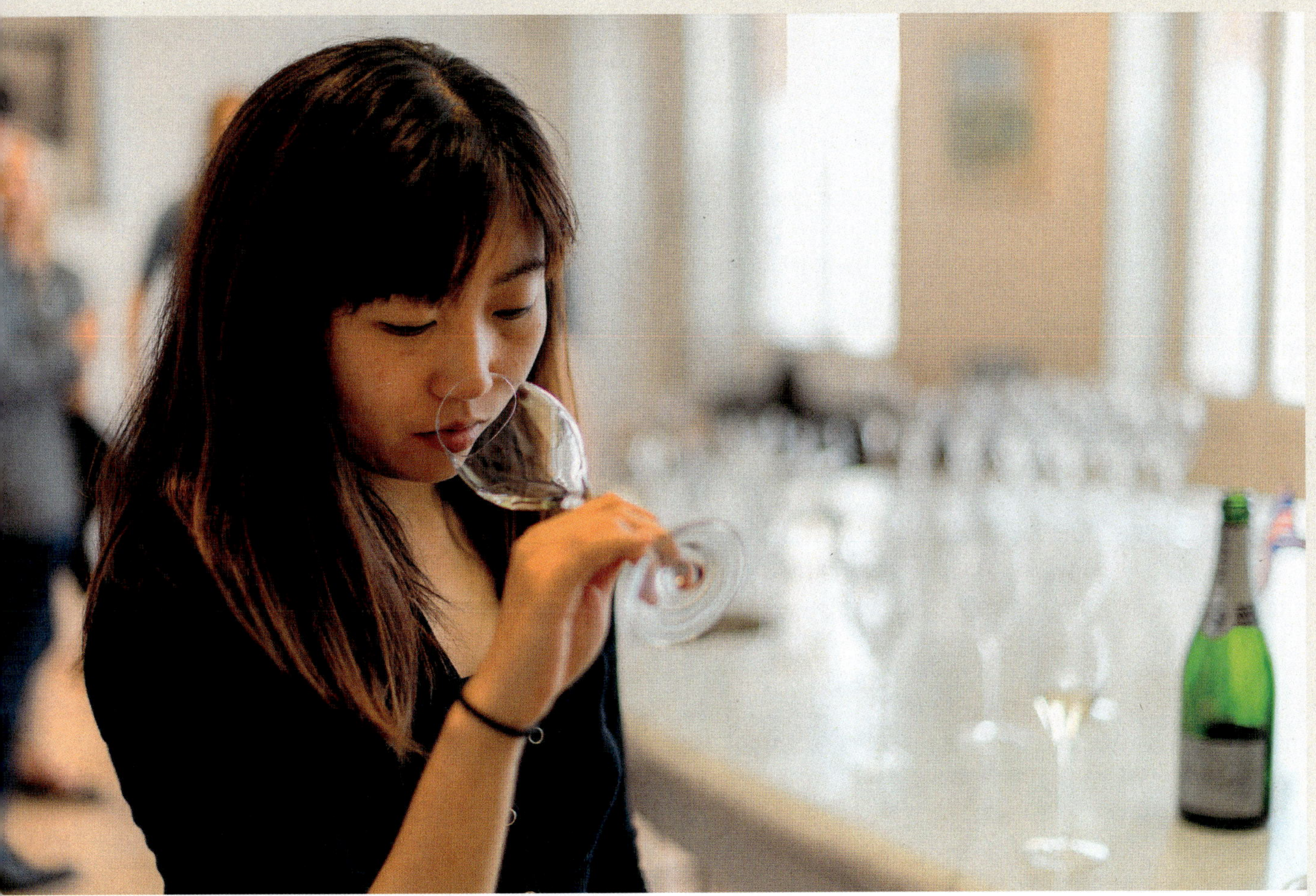

A food scientist and trained wine expert, Qian Janice Wang loves flavor. An avid dancer, she shifted her graduate research focus from music and emotion to music and food after a life-changing Michelin-starred meal. *Opposite:* A sampling of bites from a food festival Wang attended in 2019.

green-apple candy so extensible that the chefs turned it into a helium-filled balloon with a fruit-leather string. To eat it, she placed her lips on the surface of the candy and sucked in the helium.

"It really made me feel like if a three-Michelin star restaurant can play like this, then maybe there is room for doing crazy multisensory food research," Wang says. "This dinner changed my research life." She went back to MIT and switched the focus of her master's degree to music and food. It's still the most expensive meal she's ever paid for, but it was worth it. "I dedicated my master's thesis to Alinea, and I sent them a copy," she says.

It's well validated that people consider certain sounds "sweet," and that the sounds can in turn change perceptions of the true sweetness of a food, but for her latest experiment, Wang is investigating what this experience looks like in action in the brain. Her participants lie in an fMRI connected to a gustometer, which sends either sucrose or citric acid to their mouth while they listen to "sweet" or "sour" music one of Wang's graduate students composed. Then participants rate the tastes of the food. The experimental setup is complex, since the electronics that deliver the tastes would interfere with the fMRI machine: 12-meter-long tubes run from a participant's mouth in the scanner, above the ceiling, and across the walls to a separate room housing the gustometer. "If you listen to a sweet soundtrack, people rate food as tasting sweeter, and if you listen to a sour soundtrack, the food tastes more sour," Wang says. "But this would be the first time that we see what the neural response is, and for me this is so exciting."

Swiftsure Regatta, a series of weekend yacht races that course through the Strait of Juan de Fuca, the geographical border between her home on Vancouver Island and Washington State in the United States. At the regatta parties, Small, new to alcohol at the time, had an all too relatable run-in with coconut-flavored rum cloaked beneath syrupy soda. In the end, she got sick.

"To this day, I will not drink a Malibu and Seven-Up," says Small. "However, in the ensuing 30 years, I didn't develop an aversion to sweet things, I formed an aversion to the exact thing that made me sick. That's the value of flavor, which is hugely important in terms of adaptation." Without flavor, and only taste, this learned reaction could have pushed her to eliminate unrelated sweet foods from her diet that provide sources of nutrients and energy needed for survival, such as bananas or milk.

RODENTS HAVE A totally different pathway from food to brain than the one humans and nonhuman primates share; the latter pathway may make this specialized aversion experience possible. In rodents, signals localized to the mouth move into the brainstem, and then split at the pons: One pathway goes to the amygdala, and then the hypothalamus; the other pathway goes to the thalamus, the insula, and then the primary taste cortex. This means that the sensory experience of taste and the salience of eating are disconnected. In primate brains, there is no such split. Instead, information moves from the mouth, to the brainstem, skips the pons altogether, and goes straight into the thalamus, the brain's switchboard. Sensory and emotional experiences around food are processed together.

MANIPULATING THE MIND

A CUP OF coffee seems so simple: roasted beans, steeped in hot water. But there's vast room for customizing how we drink it that shows how interconnected the brain's experience of food is. Try a sip of your morning coffee unadulterated. The dominant taste will be bitter. Now, add a teaspoon of sugar and try again.

"[The sugar] didn't change how much bitterness was in there from a chemical perspective, but it changed how much bitterness was there from a sensory perspective," says Dando, the Cornell food scientist. Throughout the

The brain consistently associates certain colors, shapes, sounds, and tastes without us necessarily being aware. In studies, most people assign the sharp shape, made from cheese, to the nonsense word "kiki," and the rounded shape, made from chocolate syrup, to "bouba."

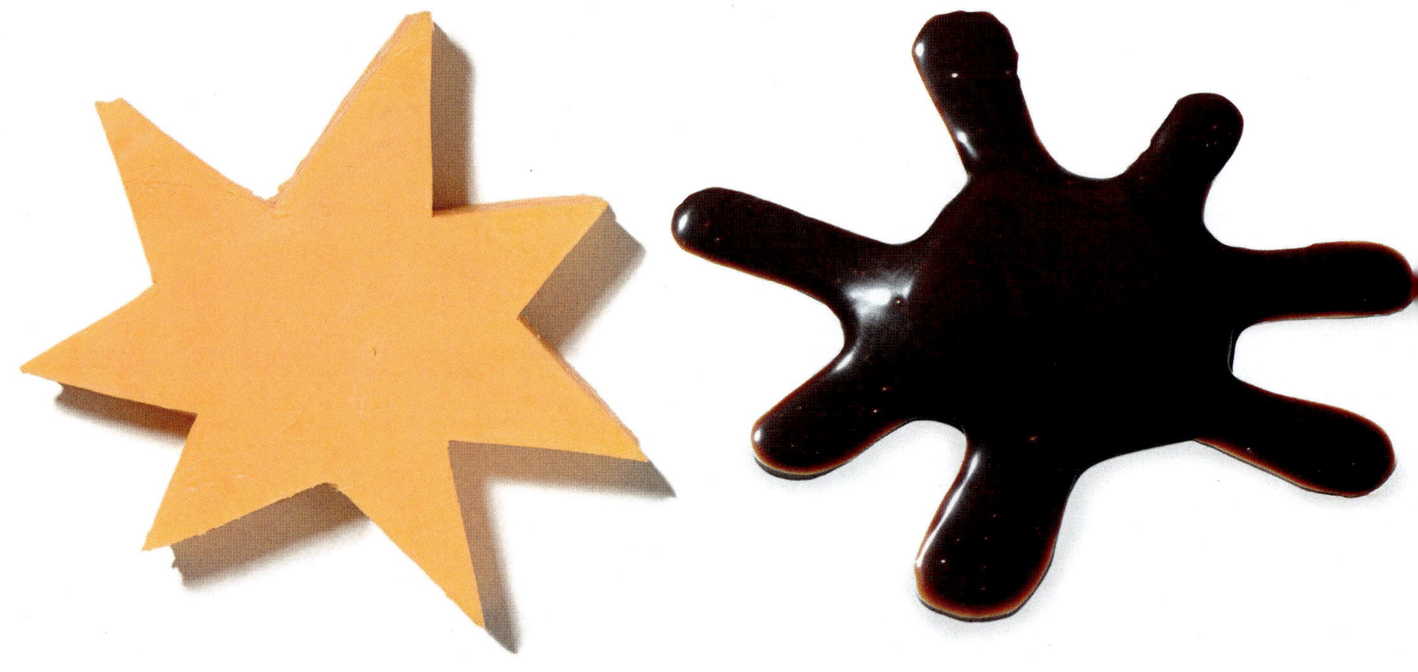

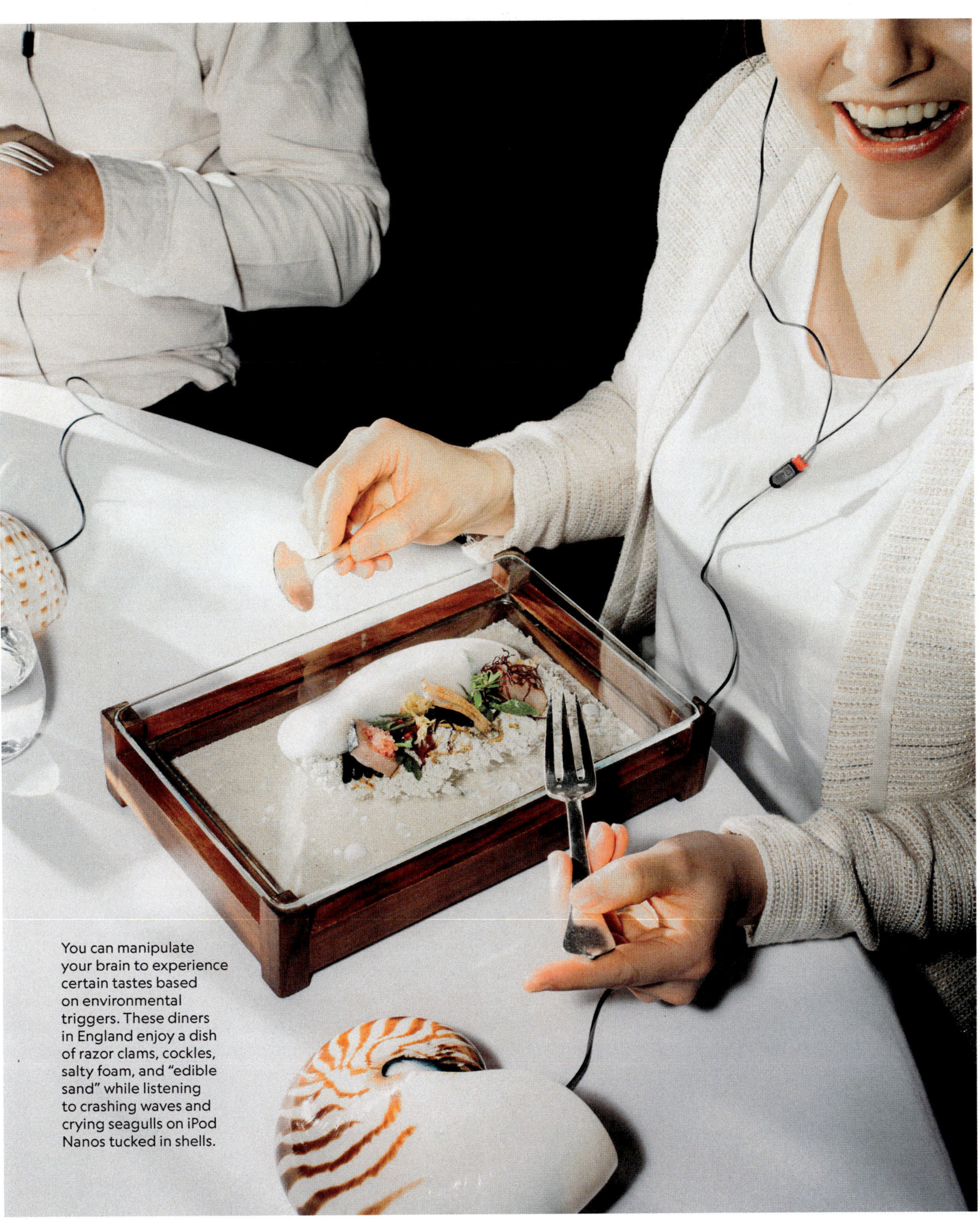

You can manipulate your brain to experience certain tastes based on environmental triggers. These diners in England enjoy a dish of razor clams, cockles, salty foam, and "edible sand" while listening to crashing waves and crying seagulls on iPod Nanos tucked in shells.

day, you can play with ingredients like this on a grander, more flavorful scale: For dinner, try sautéing mushrooms in butter, and then deglaze the pan with a splash of pickle juice—you won't perceive the pickle juice, but the mushrooms will taste more mushroom-y. For dessert, make a chocolate cake with a dash of hot coffee in the batter. The end result isn't something that you'd describe as mocha, but rather an exceptionally chocolate-y cake.

For the flavor researchers who incorporate vision and hearing into the equation, experimentally manipulating this complex system—and expectations around food—is a huge source of intrigue. In one experiment, Wang asks her participants to drink their coffee with a virtual reality headset obscuring their vision. As each person lifts a real mug of coffee to their mouth, they see an identical mug of coffee move in tandem in virtual space. This blended experience is called augmented virtuality, and it's how Wang pushes the visual system's manipulation of flavor experiences to its outer limits.

The coffee participants drink in real life is without cream—or sugar, for that matter—but Wang can alter the coffee they see moving toward them in virtual space to visually appear as though it has cream in it. Users who see a lighter-colored coffee in virtual space report the coffee they drink in reality seems creamier than it does when the virtual coffee also appears to be black.

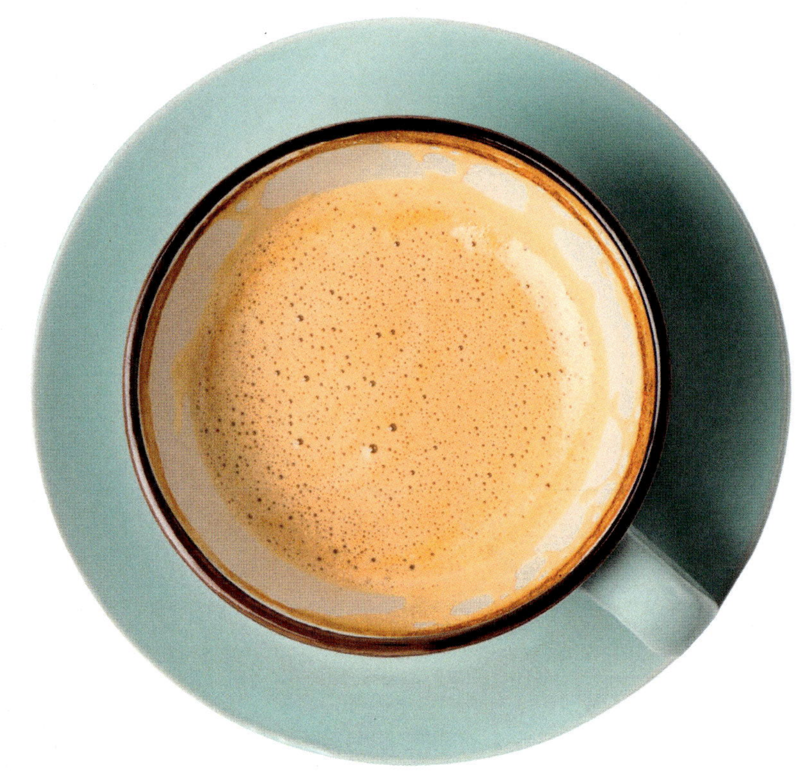

Researchers have found that lighter-colored coffee can fool the brain into perceiving a creamy flavor whether or not cream is present.

> **Unlike other senses, such as vision, you can train your brain to get better at smell and taste, enhancing the experience and joy of flavor.**

FOR DECADES, SCIENTISTS have known that color changes perceptions about flavor, but it's only been possible to test in certain kinds of foods, such as adding a red dye to chardonnay to trick people into perceiving it as having the flavor of a rosé. But until now, there has never been an easy way to test whether this same principle holds for something with physical properties like coffee, where dye wouldn't show up.

Because flavor is such a nuanced system, it's not clear that this ability to manipulate it experimentally could ever have any real-world effect on diet. It's unlikely we'll be tricking our brains into experiencing a low-fat food as being perfectly delicious anytime soon. But using what scientists know about flavor to manipulate the less complex taste system is a more realistic possibility. For example, you can reduce the sugar content of a beverage and augment it with other "sweet" cues, such as an added strawberry or caramel aroma, to trick the brain into thinking sugar is there.

A growing body of research also indicates that altering someone's environment changes the outcome of taste. Beyond adding a tricky aroma to a sugar-free beverage, you might go many steps further to induce the false experience of sweetness by dyeing the drink pink, and serving it in a round cup, in a pink room, while high-pitched chimes tinkle in the background. It's an exaggerated example, but these are just some of the many external factors—colors, shapes, and sounds—that can increase someone's sensation of sweetness.

Although the basis for these robust systems of experiencing food are primarily there to help us seek out nutrients, avoid toxins, and eat until we're full without going too far, the modern experience of food is something more. It's about culture, memory, wonderment, and learning. "Flavor is really interesting because if you train, you do get better," Wang says, of detecting nuances in what we eat and drink, and deriving joy from the experience. Other senses are more fixed. For example, you can't train yourself out of nearsightedness, only surgery can correct that. But because smell and taste neurons regenerate every few weeks, there are opportunities to master experiencing flavor at new heights. "These are things in our bodies [that], even when we're adults, we can still make better, and that's so cool," says Wang.

Qian Janice Wang is running a study in which participants taste coffee in virtual reality to see how much its color impacts flavor.

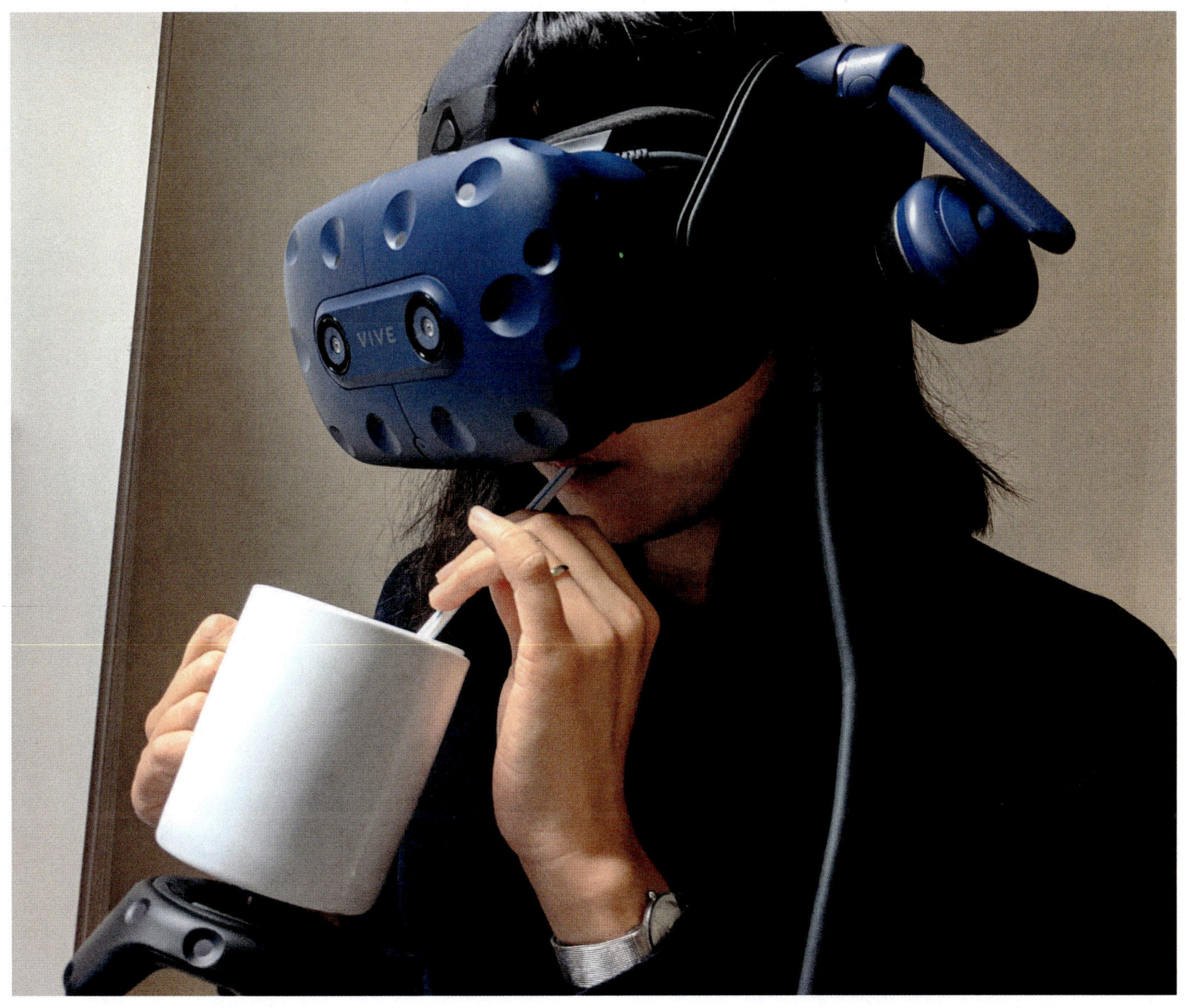

CHAPTER 3

HURT BRAINS HURT PEOPLE

Brain injury and chronic pain reshape how the brain works, and yet the brain itself can't feel pain.

Pain is one of the most unpleasant parts of being alive, there's no way to sugarcoat it. Yet it's also one of the most important. Physical pain is a critical language the body speaks to tell the brain about danger in your environment. The brain, in turn, mediates your behavior to keep you safe. Without pain, you'd leave your hand on a hot stove forever, and burn off all your skin. This back-and-forth communication between body and brain isn't foolproof, though. Some people's brains go too far, keeping the communication on high alert even when the threat has dissipated, or the injury has healed.

"Acute pain usually has a purpose, a good purpose: to alert you that something is going on, and possibly to remove yourself from that situation," says Karen Davis, head of brain, imaging, and behavior at the Krembil Brain Institute in Toronto, Canada. "It's thought that once [pain] becomes chronic, it may not serve any purpose anymore."

Chronic pain is diagnosed as pain that lasts more than three to six months and is seemingly untethered from any physical trauma. It's no longer sending useful messages that can aid in healing and safety. When people who live with chronic pain visit clinicians trained to look for obvious signs of injury, they are often brushed off and told the pain is "all in their head." While these comments all too often make patients feel unheard at best or gaslit at worst, there

The experience of bodily pain is a subjective one that starts and ends with the brain, even though the brain itself cannot feel pain. Researchers are increasingly looking to understand how the complex pain network functions, so they can better ease it without opioids.

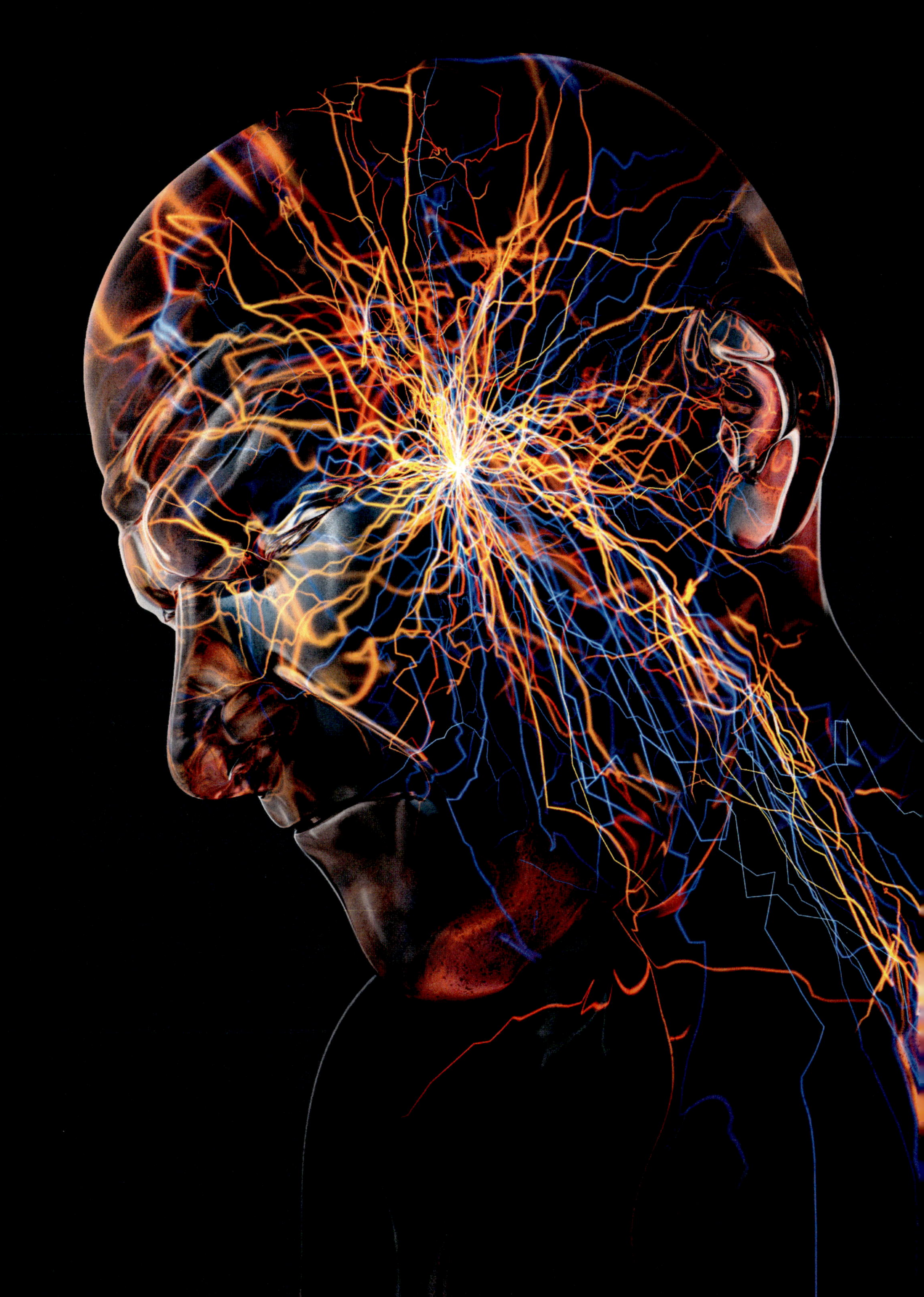

is an unintentional element of truth behind the dismissive phrase. The very real pain they feel lurking around the edges of medical understanding does start and end in the brain.

The World Health Organization estimates that one in 10 adults are newly diagnosed with chronic pain each year, making the call for targeted treatments an urgent public health issue. But because both acute and chronic pain travel the same pathways to the brain, those who hunt for treatments for the latter walk an incredibly fine line: How do you shut off unnecessary chronic pain without shutting off necessary acute pain, such as the feeling of a bee sting? Because the brain has neither a designated pain center nor can it feel pain inside itself, the way our other body parts can, researchers instead focus on understanding why the communication system about bodily injuries sometimes misfires, and how internal brain injuries work.

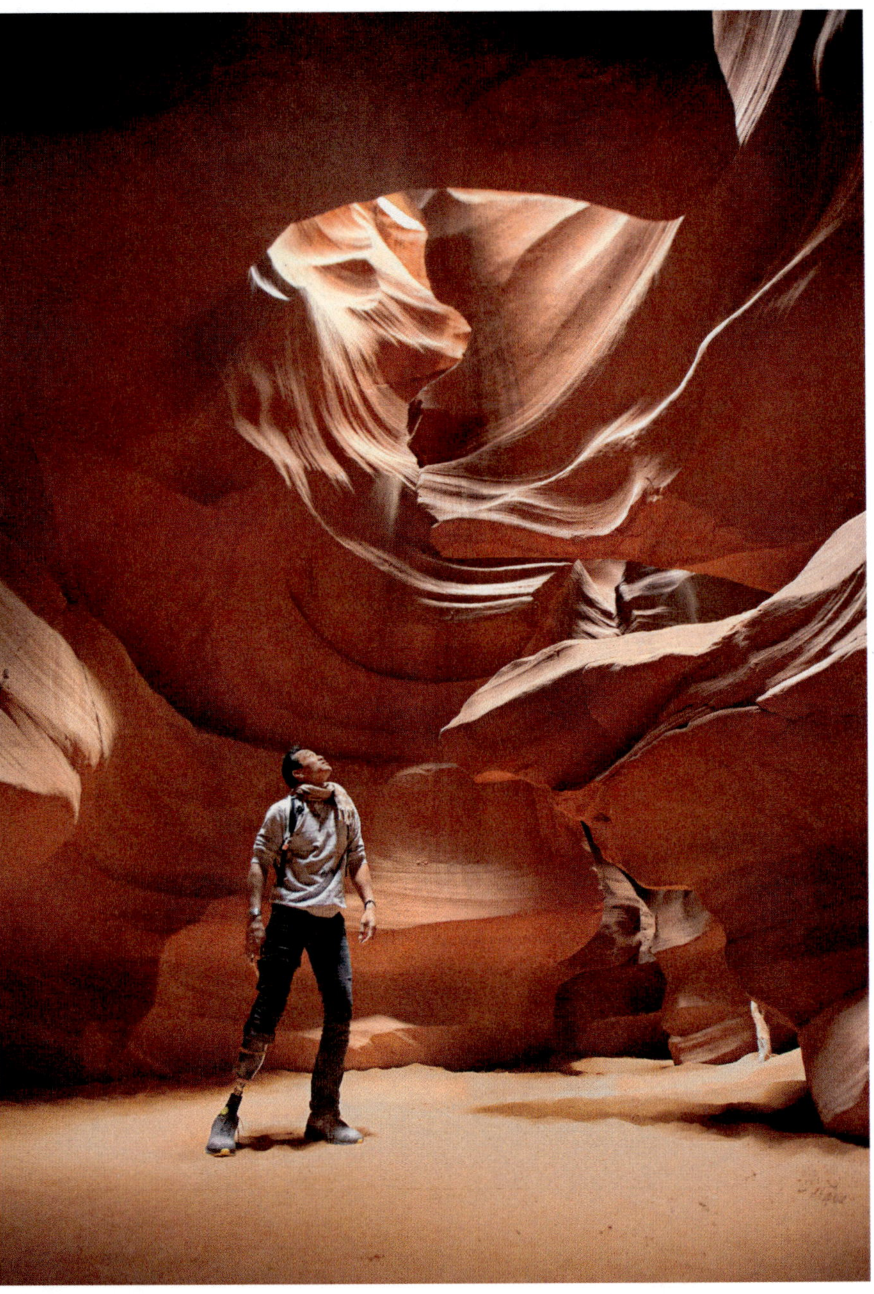

"What I learned in my physical experience is that so much of my reality is defined entirely in my mind," says Albert Lin, a National Geographic Explorer who began searching for alternative forms of therapy for pain after undergoing an amputation.

ALL IN YOUR HEAD

SAY THE WORD "pain" and the first thing that may come to mind is probably some sort of physical agony—perhaps the swift slice of a paper cut or the more diffuse throbbing of a burn. But these complex experiences actually have two crude biological levels, one of which is painless, in a way. When sharp paper first breaks the skin on your finger, nerve cells in the body send alert signals to the brain that something terrible is happening. The brain, in turn, quickly problem solves, instructing the body to activate inflammation to stop the trauma and begin the healing process.

But this is not pain exactly; it is what's called nociception. Just because a brain scan shows neural activity that seems to be related to physical trauma "doesn't necessarily mean that somebody is feeling pain," Davis says. While under anesthesia, for example, a brain scan would show you were having a nociceptive response to surgical trauma, but while unconscious, you're not in pain, per se. Pain is the cognitive blanket over the whole experience: your ability to intricately put words to a physical adversary as though it were as nuanced as flavor—something sharp or dull—and as subjective.

"The interesting part of all this is that no two people have the same response to the same injury—or surgery, for that matter," says Akiko Okifuji, professor of pain medicine at the University of Utah. "Two people may undergo exactly the same procedure, but they may come up with a very different pain response and also [pain relief] requirements."

EMOTIONAL PAIN MAY even play a role in your subjective experience of physical pain. In 2012, a review in *Nature* of a few pain studies concluded that both physical and emotional pain follow similar neural pathways. According to the review, social rejection activated the dorsal anterior cingulate cortex and anterior insula, the same areas active in physical pain, as did "experiences of negative social evaluation, rejection from a romantic partner, and bereavement."

The year after this review came out, Anne Leppert, then 37, visited the Pain Management Center at University of Utah Health for the first time after enduring financial distress, the end of a romantic relationship, and the loss of her grandmother back-to-back. Through it all, only an unrelenting pain—without any related physical injury—stood by her side. After a year

Two people may undergo exactly the same procedure, but they may experience very different pain responses.

Pain is subjective. During surgery, a brain scan would show you were having a nociceptive response, but while unconscious under anesthesia, you're not in pain per se.

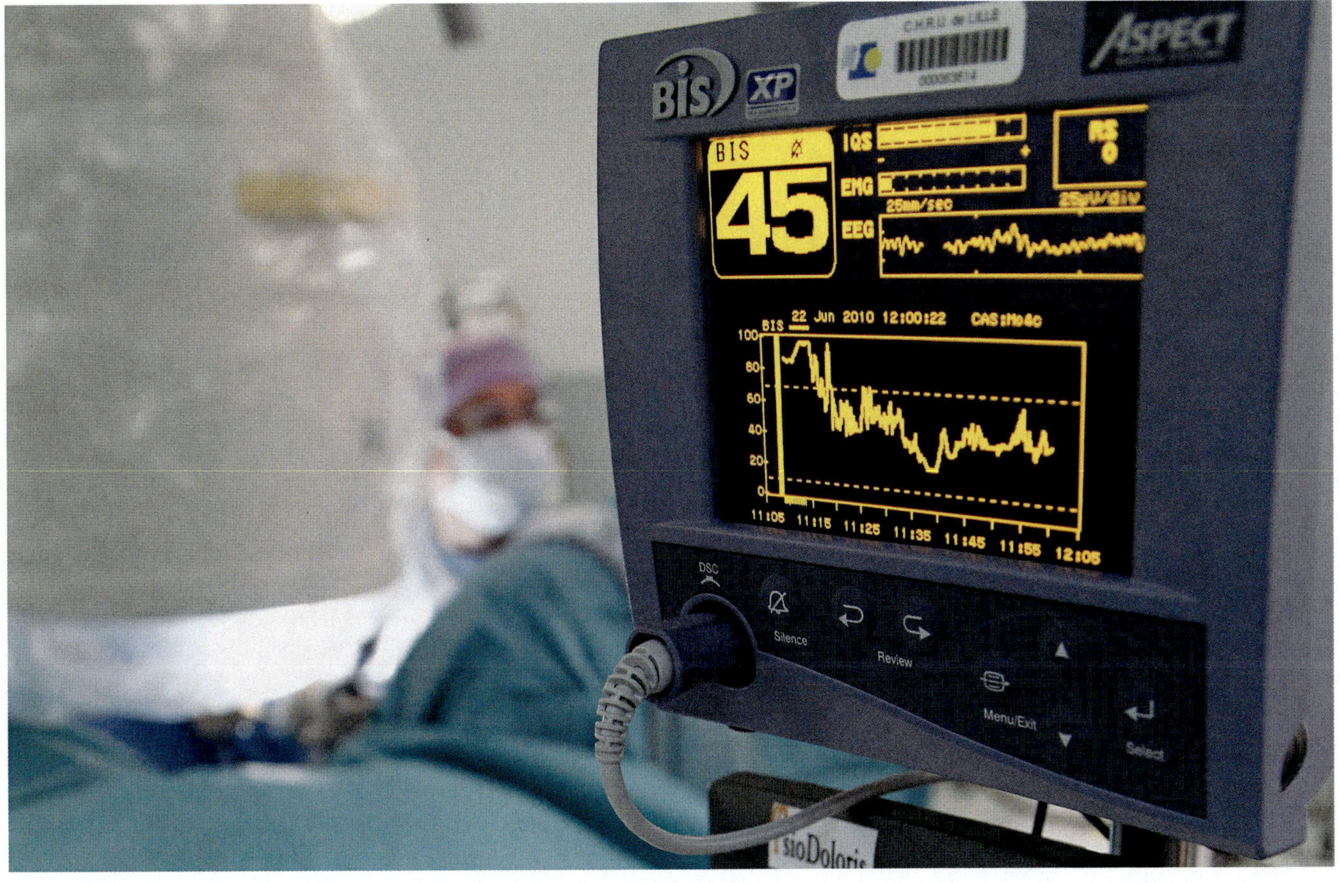

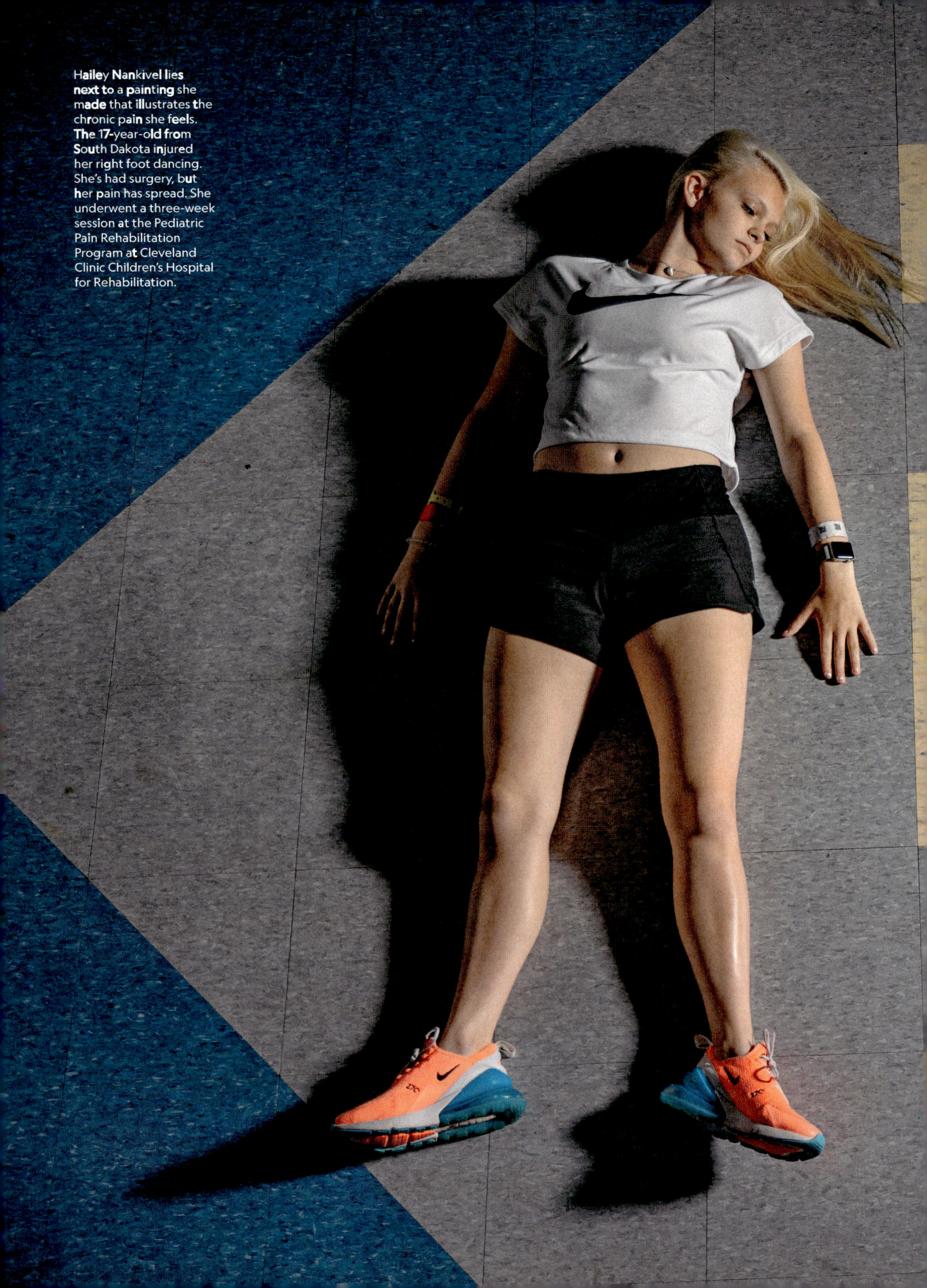

Hailey Nankivel lies next to a painting she made that illustrates the chronic pain she feels. The 17-year-old from South Dakota injured her right foot dancing. She's had surgery, but her pain has spread. She underwent a three-week session at the Pediatric Pain Rehabilitation Program at Cleveland Clinic Children's Hospital for Rehabilitation.

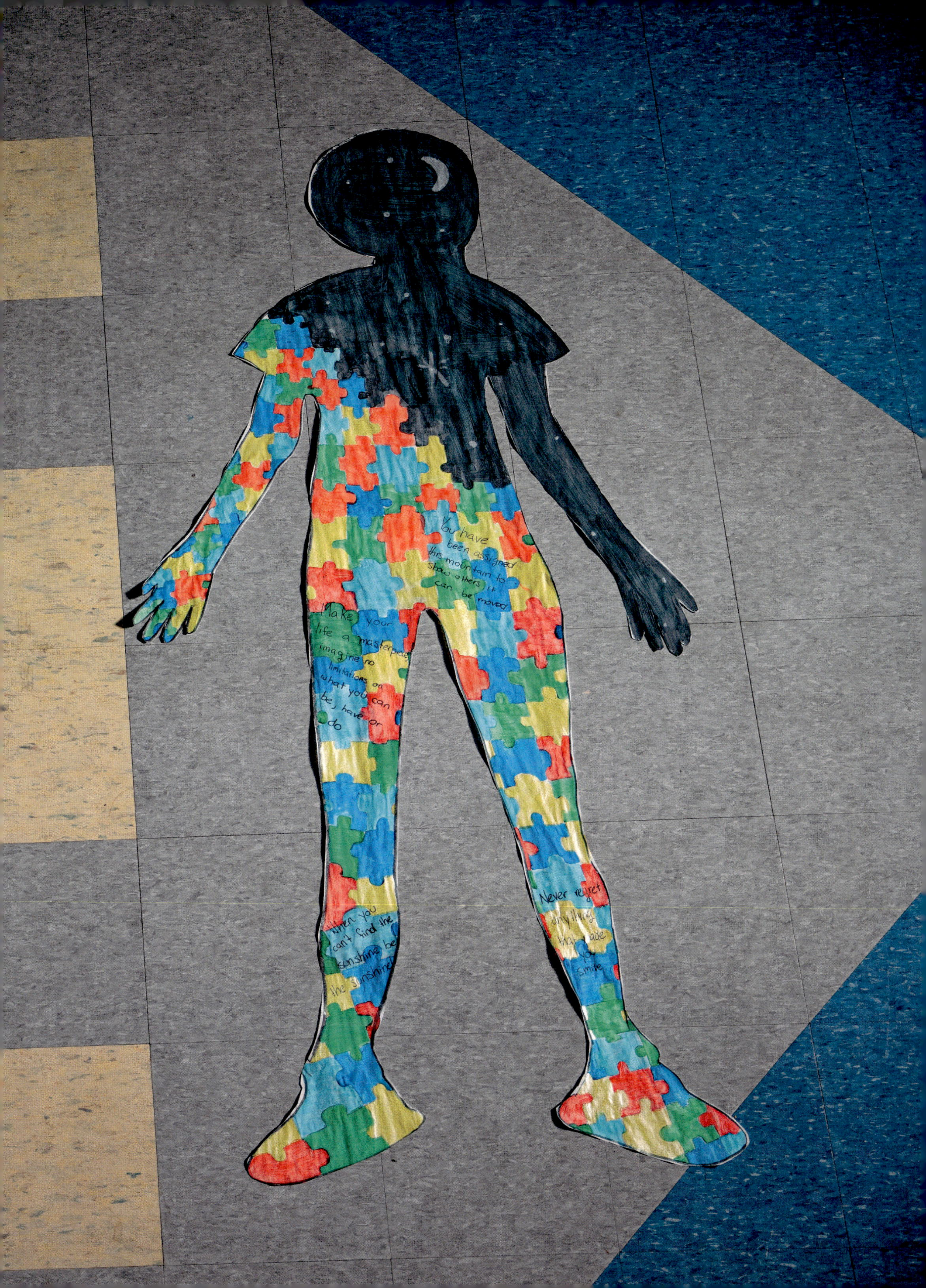
You have been assigned this mountain to show others it can be moved
Make your life a masterpiece imagine no limitations on what you can be, have or do
When you can't find the sonshine be the sunshine
Never regret anything that ade you smile

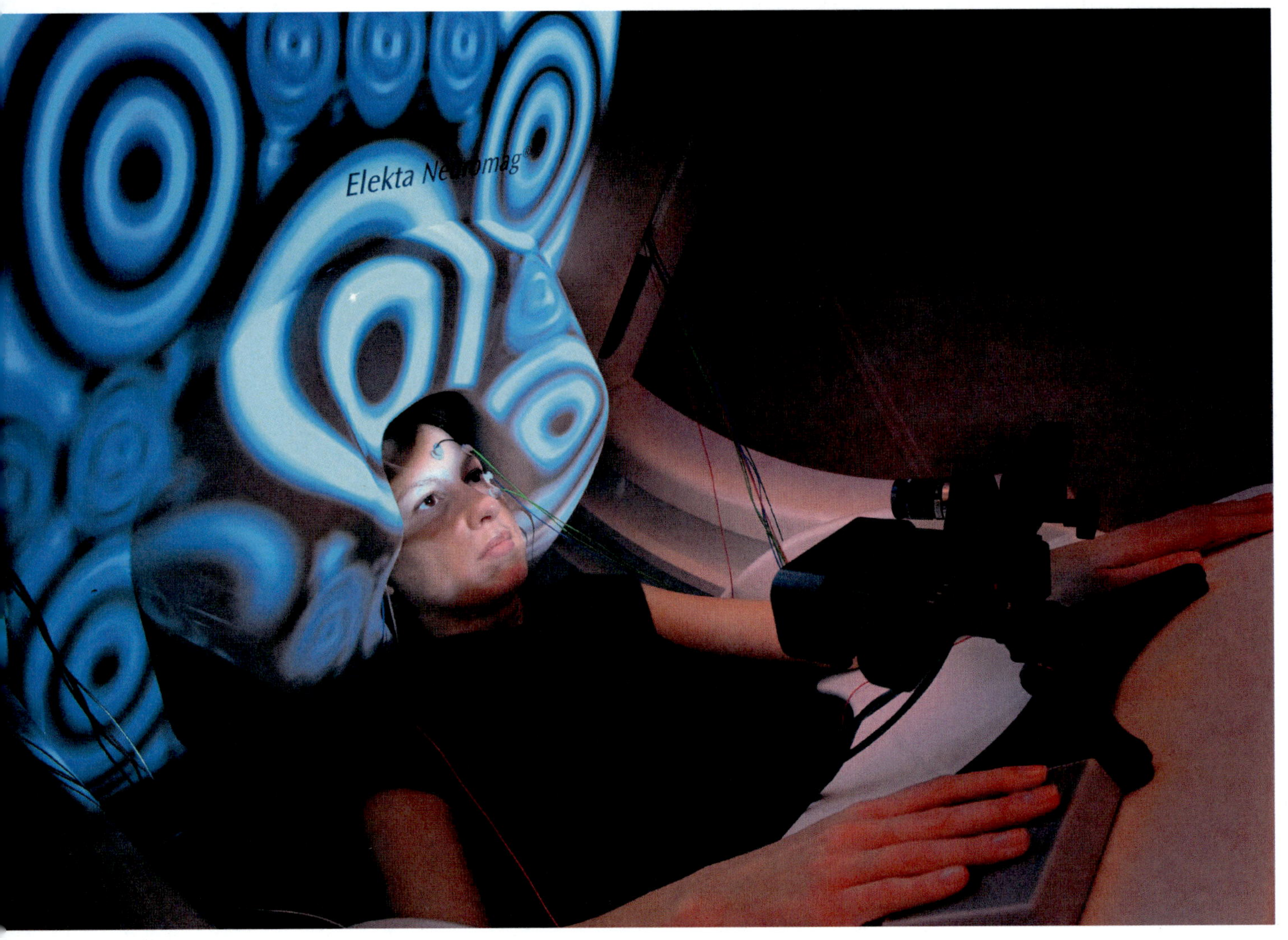

Noninvasive imaging tools are key to better understanding the brain in pain since surgical access to the brain is so intense and risky. Up-and-coming magnetoencephalography (MEG), shown here, seems to blend the best of existing tools like EEG and fMRI.

of feeling this unexplained sensation, she wanted answers. When seated, a burning sensation moved up Leppert's spine and radiated across her back, reaching out to other areas of her body "like a current." For years prior, she had lived with chronic fatigue syndrome and a fluctuating achy feeling, also in her back, but it was manageable enough for her to rock climb, whitewater raft, hike, and ski. She knew something was different about this burning, and that she needed medical intervention. The center she visited is partly a research institution, designed to help sleuth for explanations of unexplained pain, but not to treat patients long-term. After two years, Leppert's doctors discharged her with diagnoses of generalized pain disorder, central pain disorder, and pain amplification syndrome (a new term for fibromyalgia).

After her discharge from the pain center, she mostly saw physicians with little specialized knowledge of her conditions and fought bitterly to receive Social Security disability benefits from the U.S. government.

The stress of feeling undermined while navigating both of these systems correlated with an even worse return of the burning pain: this time in other parts of her body, even her legs. "The intensity was such that I couldn't even sit down, so I knew I needed more help," Leppert says. She approached the Pain Management Center again, unsure if she'd be allowed back. But Okifuji, who also does clinical work there, took her on, knowing all too well how often the chronic pain of women and minorities is dismissed by people who don't understand pain without obvious injury. "I hear that a lot," Okifuji says. "Their pain is real, and we just don't understand everything about it."

IMAGING THE BRAIN

BEING ABLE TO "get inside" the brain with imaging tools such as MRI and fMRI has been a boon for neuroscientists, who historically have only been able to understand the live, active brain with risky surgical invasion. Although groundbreaking, these giant magnetic machines that require special shielded rooms are still expensive to buy and operate, which holds back underfunded neuroscience research.

"Chronic pain is one of the most expensive, and probably one of the most debilitating, conditions, yet the funding . . . is disproportionately small," says Okifuji. "I hate to talk about money, but that does have an impact on how much you can do in terms of science."

Davis, the researcher in Toronto, is hopeful that within a few years, an

In an MRI study at the University of Maryland, Baltimore scientists trained subjects to perceive a heat stimulus as hotter when they saw a face in distress at the same time.

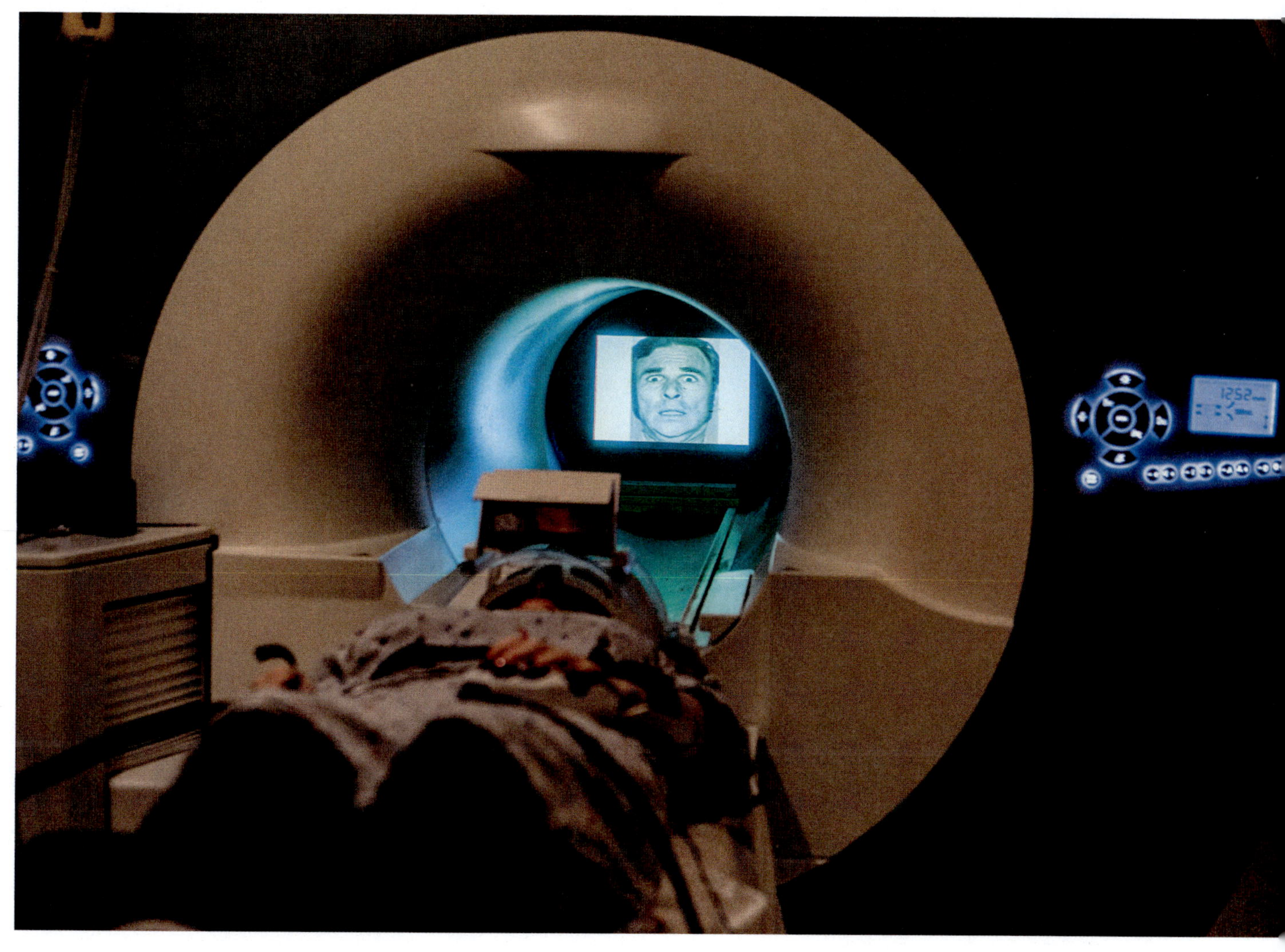

THE REWARD CIRCUIT

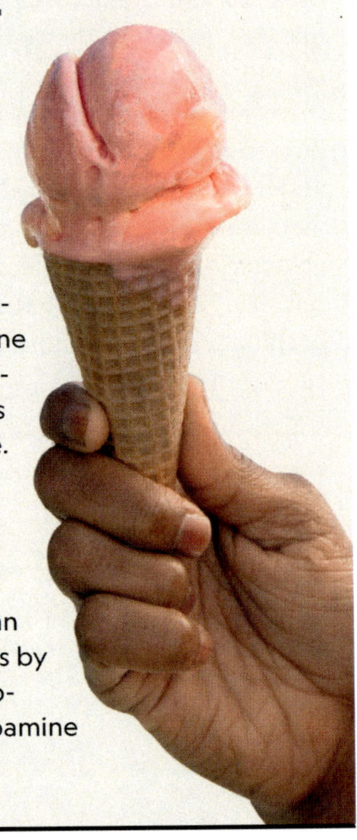

One of the oldest pathways in the brain is also among the most intractable: the reward circuit, responsible for everything from moderate feelings of joy to full-blown addiction. Its gateway is the brain's ventral tegmental area, first seen in vertebrates 500 million years ago. Neurons, after passing through this gateway, send information about rewarding experiences into the brain's nucleus accumbens by expelling dopamine—a type of chemical called a neurotransmitter that neurons release and absorb to communicate. The nucleus accumbens is a highly connected area of the brain with tentacles in the limbic system, the brain's ancient emotional center, and in the prefrontal cortex, which controls executive functioning, such as decision-making. When an activity ignites this complex pathway, the outcome is the brain creating positive associations, encouraging us to seek out, or even crave, the behavior again.

What makes the difference between enjoying a glass of wine and being an alcoholic is partly related to how much dopamine is hanging out between neurons at any time. The brain keeps a fine balance on this because, for example, too little dopamine can develop into Parkinson's disease and too much dopamine can lead to addiction. Dopamine that's just right evokes healthy feelings of pleasure.

Addictive drugs are exceptionally good at tipping this balance: some by encouraging neurons to release more dopamine than they normally would, others by blocking neurons from reabsorbing it, keeping the dopamine in free flow.

up-and-coming imaging tool called MEG—magnetoencephalography—can make some of this noninvasive work more accessible and robust. An fMRI scan shows spatial activity in the brain, but indirectly: The activation of neurons increases oxygen in blood flowing nearby, and it's that oxygenation that fMRI captures. An EEG test, which relies on a skullcap covered in electrodes, is far less expensive to run, and represents electrical information that comes directly from neurons. But the drawback of EEG is that it can only show you what neurons are doing over time, not where in the brain the activity is coming from. A MEG image blends the best of both tools, picking up activity directly from neurons over time and offering information about which brain regions this activity occurs in.

> **Pain is an interconnected experience that recruits many areas of the brain, including busy cortical regions responsible for memory and emotion.**

BUT EVEN THE best imaging tools will still run into the simple problem that there is no single brain region that generates pain. Pain is an interconnected experience that recruits many different areas of the brain, including busy cortical regions responsible for memory and emotion. These regions may be engaged in other activities while also giving rise to pain. A person can be in pain while learning a new language or listening to music, and it would be impossible to tell which experience brain activity is tied to. Finding pain in the brain "is almost like a needle in a haystack," Davis says. "We're looking at a small amount of what else is going on."

Instead, personalized treatments for chronic pain are more likely to come from a better understanding of the individual molecular pathways that mediate pain perception. Such pathways could also provide telltale pretreatment clues about who would benefit most from which treatments. Davis was senior author of a related small experiment in 2018 that investigated how one might predict who would benefit from low-dose ketamine treatments for chronic pain.

Ketamine is a drug most often used clinically as an anesthetic. It blocks NMDA receptors in the brain and disrupts nociception—the communication to the brain about bodily trauma. But at uncontrolled, recreational doses, ketamine is also a powerful psychedelic drug. In the study, Davis and her team carefully monitored dosage to hit the sweet spot of blocking pain communication without knocking a person unconscious or inducing trippy imagery. Only half the participants in the study ended up benefiting from the drug, but all participants within the successful half had two crucial things in common: Imaging taken before treatment showed the default network in their brains—a network of brain areas that deal with cognition—was more connected to the nociceptive communication pathway leaving the brain than those who didn't benefit from ketamine. And behavioral tests showed that those who benefitted also had a malfunctioning perception of pain over time.

A normal response to repeated pinpricks is the feeling of pain mounting as the pinpricks progress. Participants in the study who did *not* have this typical response turned out to be those whose chronic pain responded well to ketamine. Having a behavioral test that can predict successful pain treatment is huge. Such tools would make it easier, faster, and cheaper to implement personalized pain treatments than imaging will ever be able to. But these kinds of approaches are still highly experimental, and for folks like Leppert who are currently living with and navigating their chronic pain, the world can be an extremely unkind place.

Scientists are studying controlled doses of ketamine (crystals shown below) as an intriguing pain treatment. The drug blocks nociception, signals to the brain about trauma, which may misfire in those with chronic pain.

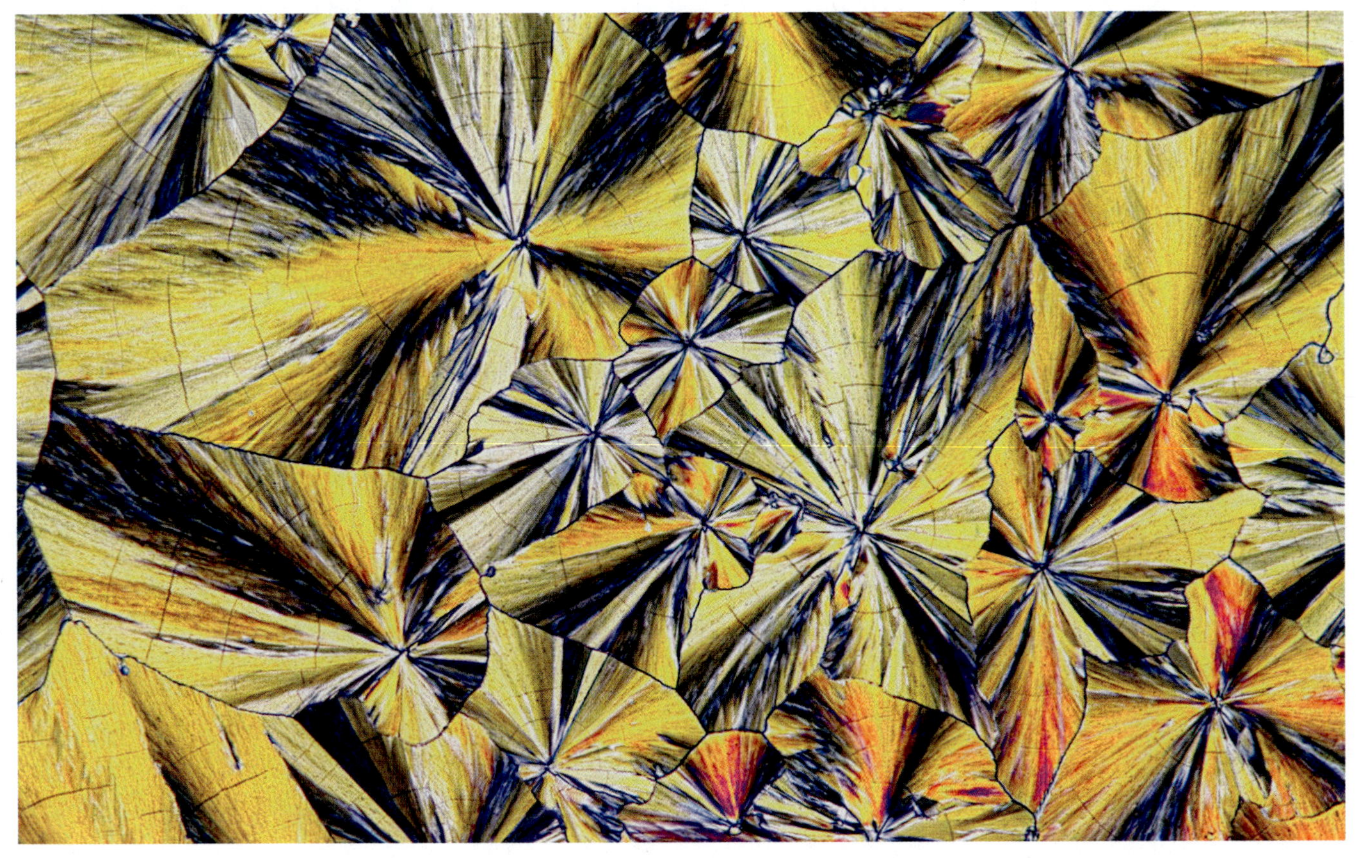

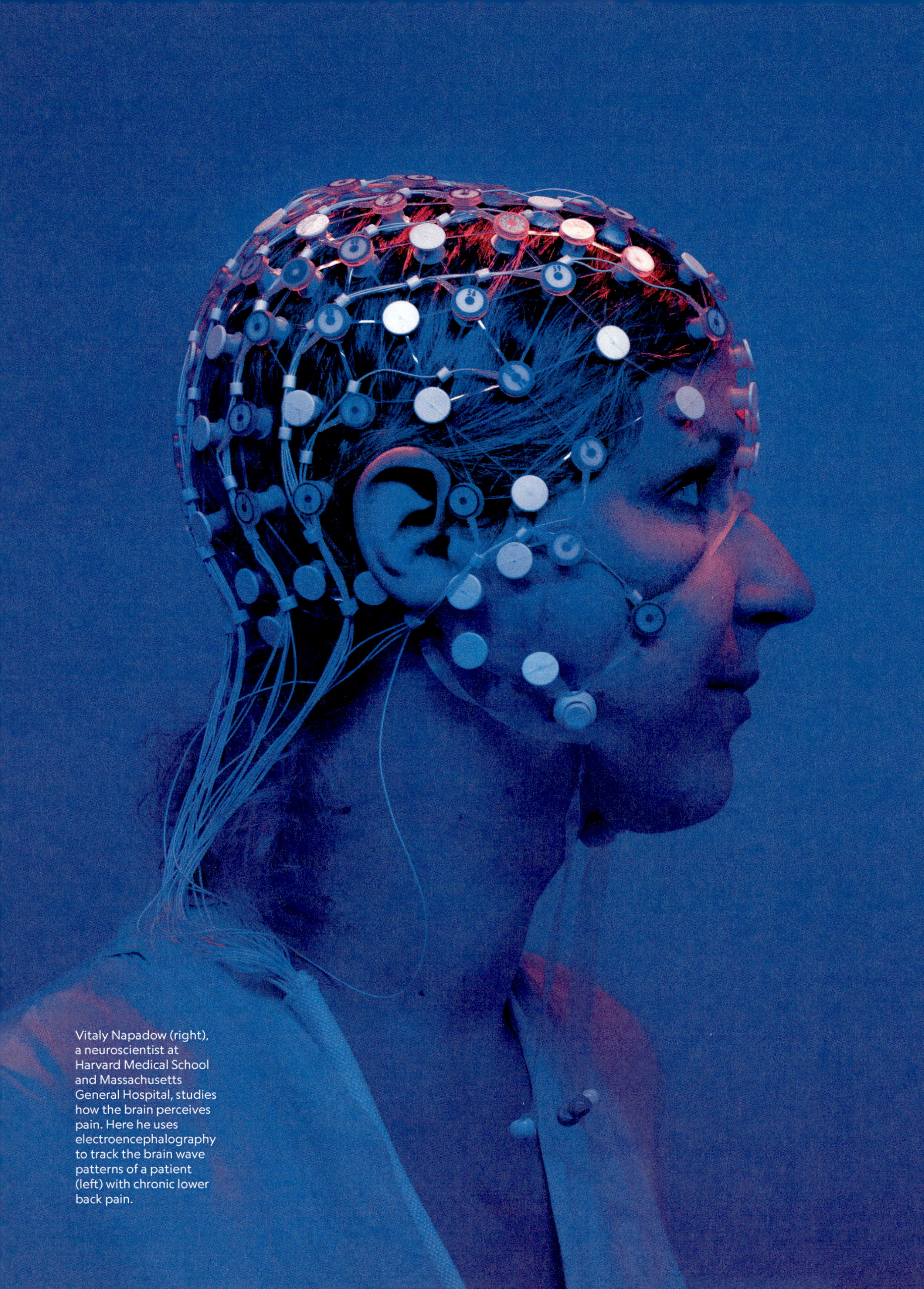

Vitaly Napadow (right), a neuroscientist at Harvard Medical School and Massachusetts General Hospital, studies how the brain perceives pain. Here he uses electroencephalography to track the brain wave patterns of a patient (left) with chronic lower back pain.

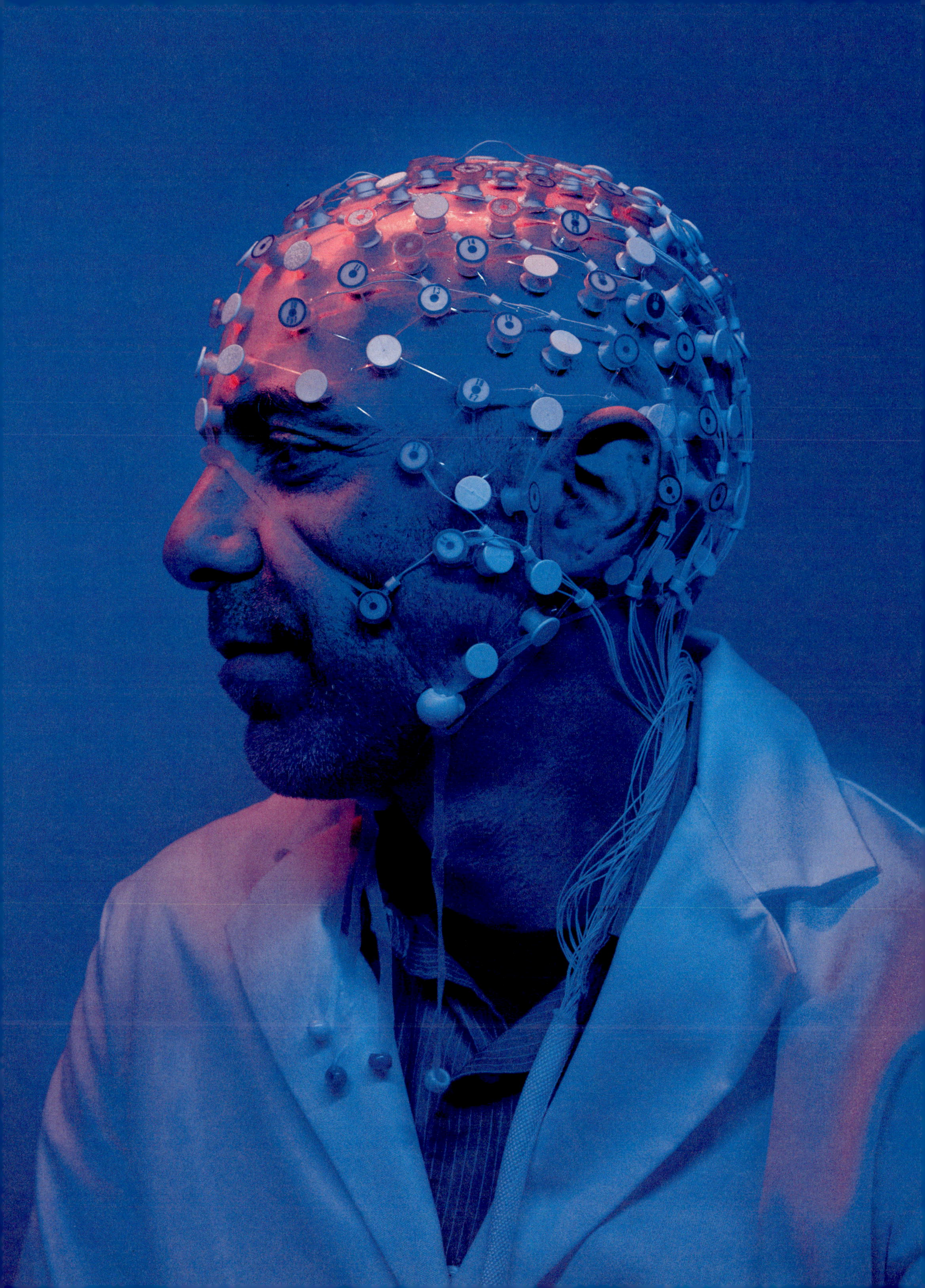

A CLOSER LOOK

GENETICALLY PAINLESS

Understanding why some people can't feel pain could yield more targeted therapies for those with chronic pain who feel too much of it.

A life without pain sounds like a dream, but in reality it can be a nightmare. Pain is a critical communication tool the body and brain use to help you safely navigate the world and learn to avoid harmful experiences in the future. The first shock of injury during a sprint might stop a runner in their tracks, leaving them with only a sprained ankle, not a broken one. It's also how we adapt: One nick from a kitchen knife, and we'll pay more attention to slicing and dicing thereafter. But a very small number of people are born with an inherited insensitivity to pain that leaves them reliant on much slower communication channels—for example, learning that their hand is touching a flame only when they smell burning skin. Broken bones and skin lesions are common among this group, who have what's called congenital analgesia.

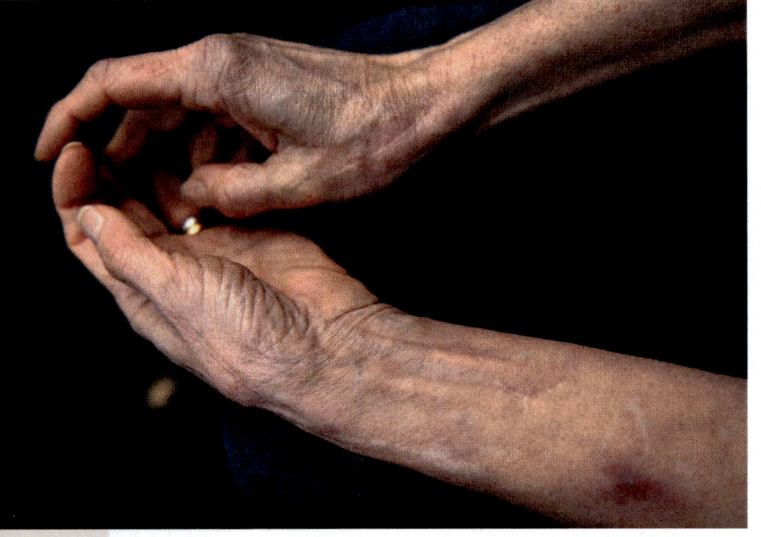

Feeling No Pain

In 2019, researchers at University College London found that a gene mutation expressed in the brain and clusters of neurons in the spinal cord underlies this faulty communication system. The gene, FAAH-OUT, normally gives rise to an enzyme that breaks down certain fatty acids. If left to proliferate, these fatty acids get in the way of not only proper nociception—the signal to the brain that a potentially painful experience is happening—but also adaptive feelings of fear-based memory and anxiety. The discovery centers on Jo Cameron, a then 71-year-old Scottish woman who acknowledged at age 65 that she had seldom felt any real pain, not even during childbirth. In her medical history, she also reported no sense of discomfort while living with osteoarthritis; only when she was nearly unable to walk did she seek out a hip replacement, at which point she had severe joint degeneration. After she opted to undergo a normally excruciating hand surgery without any pain medication, her doctors asked if she would participate in a case study.

Researchers are focused on better understanding the FAAH-OUT gene as a potential target for treating people with the opposite problem—chronic pain, which the brain continuously senses even when there is no injury. This gene is also a promising target for treating mood disorders, as its mutation confers a heightened sense of joy and optimism.

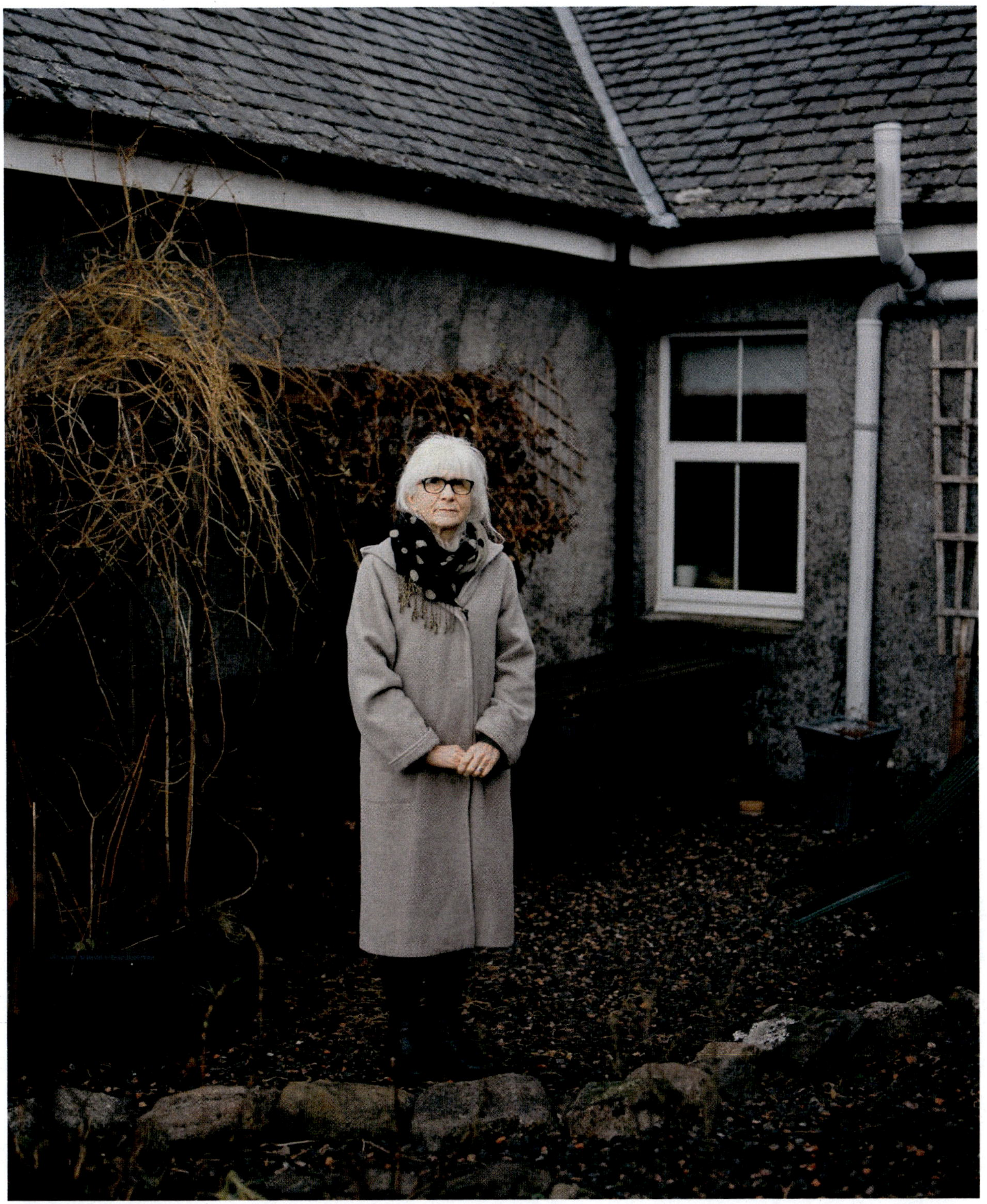

When Jo Cameron had surgery for arthritis in her hand, her anesthesiologist found she felt no pain, and referred the Scottish woman to a geneticist, who discovered she has a rare mutation. *Opposite:* Without the alert system of pain guiding their bodies, Cameron, and others like her, frequently burn their hands.

A FEW DAYS before the two of us spoke, Leppert visited a small specialty store near her house. She parked her car in a handicap spot and walked to the front door. A table of people eating lunch on a balcony above the store eyed her. "You know, that's a handicap spot," Leppert recalls one of the lunchgoers saying. "You know, we don't all look the same," Leppert shot back, wishing she had a better response. "That's the kind of typical thing I deal with because I can walk, but I can't walk a lot," she says, thinking back. The hardest part of living with chronic pain is not always the pain itself but sometimes simply its complete invisibility to other people.

Just as the person in chronic pain can seem invisible to the world, so too can the brain's own experience of injury. The headaches sometimes associated with brain trauma actually come from inflammation of the blood vessels that encase the organ. Yet the brain itself, although responsible for igniting the sensation of pain everywhere else in or on the body, doesn't turn this same perception inward.

AN UNSTOPPABLE FORCE

ANN MCKEE HAS lost track of how many human brains she's held. "Probably 3,000, not anything more than that," she says casually. Most people haven't held even one. But one of the largest collections of brains in the world lies nestled in the Boston area, and McKee is its steward.

People donate their brains to the VA-BU-CLF (UNITE) Brain Bank, which McKee founded and directs, as part of the uphill battle to understand the neurodegenerative disease called chronic traumatic encephalopathy (CTE) that arises from a series of mild blows to the head. Historically, such injuries have been brushed off as of little consequence, but McKee has been tireless—often in the face of pressure from professional sports associations, whose business would be easier if she were wrong—in showing that such trauma, if repetitive, can lead to

Cutaways of two 27-year-old brains, with the diseased brain of Aaron Hernandez, convicted murderer and tight end for the New England Patriots football team, on right. Hernandez suffered from chronic traumatic encephalopathy (CTE), the result of repeated mild hits to the head.

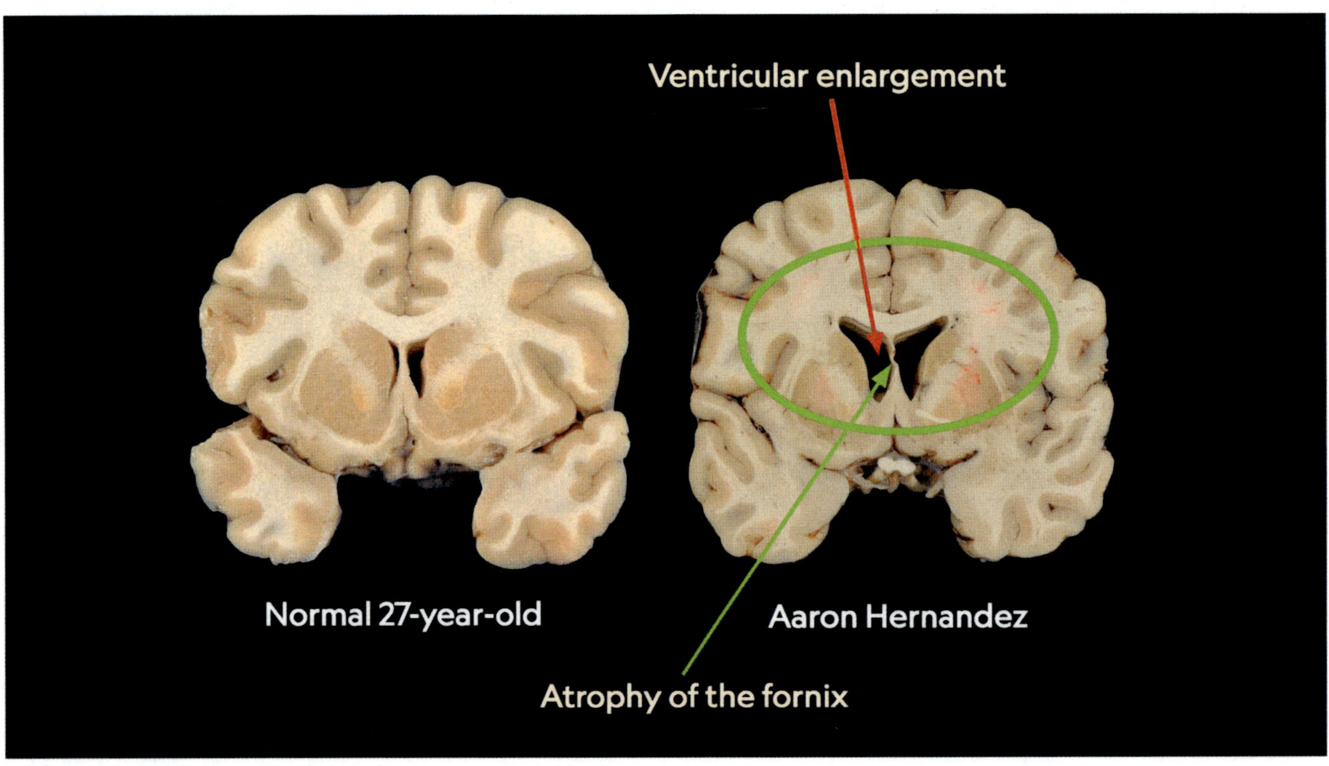

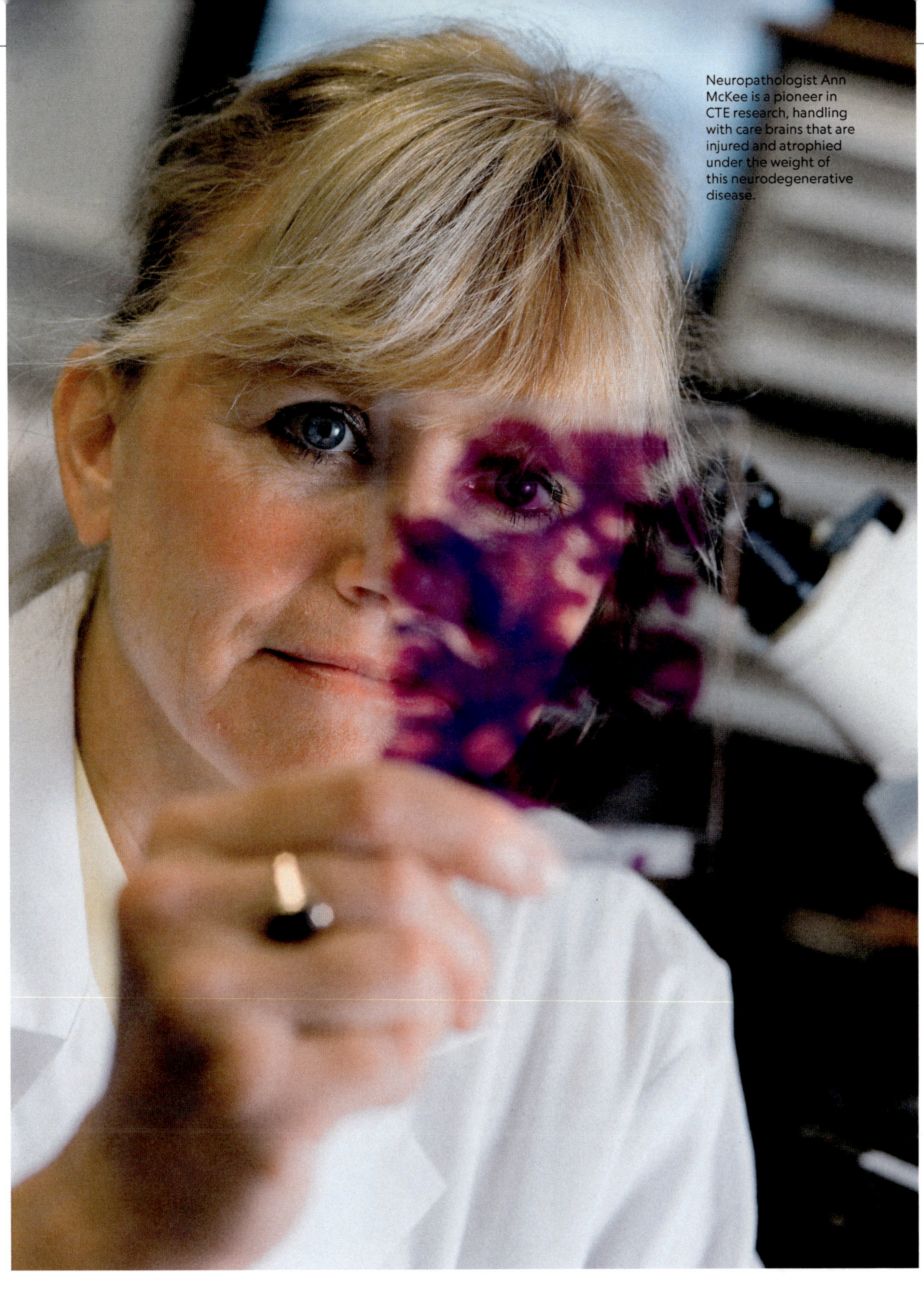

Neuropathologist Ann McKee is a pioneer in CTE research, handling with care brains that are injured and atrophied under the weight of this neurodegenerative disease.

a brain disease that keeps progressing even after the hits stop. "That whole concept is revolutionary," she says. "I am not going to hesitate to use that word."

When McKee first inspects a brain for CTE, she's looking for big signs of injury: Sometimes the corpus callosum—the structure that enables the left and right sides of the brain to communicate—is split. Often, there's damage to the frontal lobes, which handle higher-order executive functioning, and to the hippocampus, where long-term memory is stored. Altogether, the whole brain is likely shrunken. What should weigh about 49 ounces (1,400 g) is often down to about 35 ounces (1,000 g). On a microscopic level, she sees unusual patterns of tau, a protein that can be toxic to neurons. Later, she'll learn about the major personality changes witnessed by the donor's family: aggression, impulsivity, depression, memory impairment, and sometimes, ultimately, death by suicide.

BY THE TIME a brain gets to McKee, she's seeing CTE at its worst and most progressive, and after a person has already died. But it's the life of the person she's learning about through pathology that stays with her. "To look at another person's brain, to me, there's a high level

In her decades of research, Ann McKee has handled "probably 3,000" brains. In their tissue, she sees evidence of a bewildering disease.

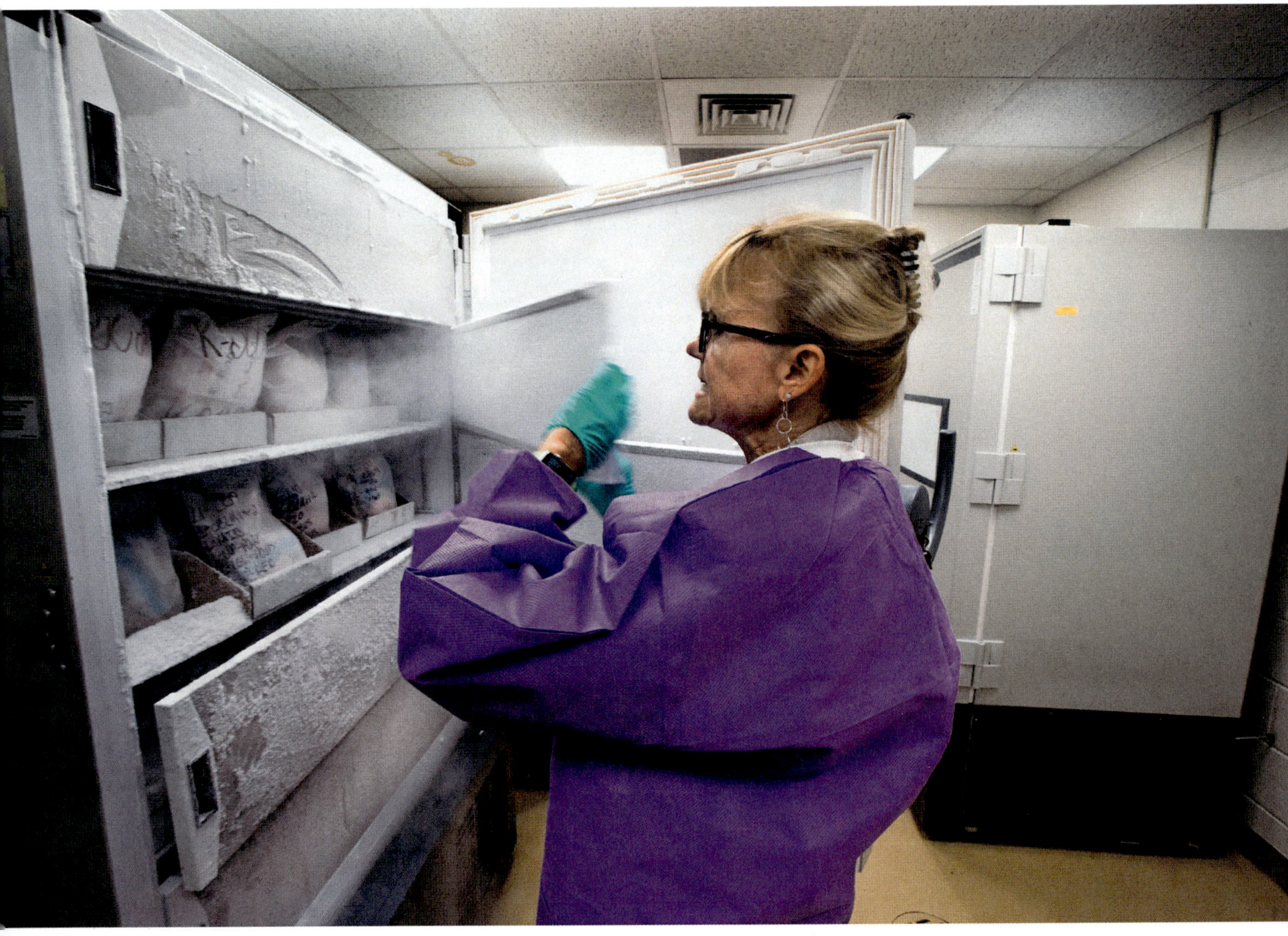

of trust and privacy," she says. "I do feel very honored in a funny way that I have this privilege."

She remembers the stories and maintains a clear visual memory of hundreds of the brains she's worked with. The best known one belonged to Aaron Hernandez, convicted murderer and tight end for the New England Patriots football team. "Just an incredible brain with tons of disease," she recalls within a millisecond.

CTE has become indelibly tied to professional football, an inconvenient reality that American sports culture can't stand, and also can't stop misunderstanding. The real takeaway is that no amount of protection from concussion will stop players from developing a disease that has nothing to do with concussions—an extreme outcome

AN ITCH YOU CAN SCRATCH

The link between the sensation of itch and the sensation of ouch is a thorny topic in neuroscience. At first blush, they appear to work through totally distinct neural pathways. You may have some instinctive understanding of this if you think about how you react to a fresh cut versus a recent mosquito bite: You wouldn't scratch the former, but you would the latter. And some classes of pain medication, such as opioids, can even cause itching as a side effect while mediating the pain response, implying some biological distinction.

But the two sensations also perplexingly share some features: They are both extreme perceptual experiences related to the sense of touch. Itch activates the same set of neurons that send bodily information to the brain about nociception—that sense of harmful stimuli that precedes a fuller cognitive perception of pain. What's more, people who are congenitally insensitive to pain also seem to be unable to perceive itch.

Scientists still have a pretty poor understanding of exactly how scratching works to abate an itch, but researchers at the Miami Itch Center found that it activates the brain's reward pathway—the same pathway triggered by eating dessert. The reward pathway not only induces feelings of pleasure but also reinforces the urge to repeat behaviors that bring about pleasure. That's why it feels impossible to stop itching poison ivy once you start—sometimes breaking through the surface of the skin to the point of bleeding—even when you know you shouldn't.

But not all itches arise from adverse experiences such as bug bites. Just as pain comes in both an acute and chronic form, so too does itch. Some people live with a persistent feeling of itch that can't be permanently abated with scratching—and that can cause them to scratch to the point of hurting themselves—that seems to arise out of nowhere. Their suffering provides the biggest incentive to better understand how pain and itch are related. If the two do indeed have overlapping pathways, perhaps validated treatments that help with pain could someday be used to stop chronic itch.

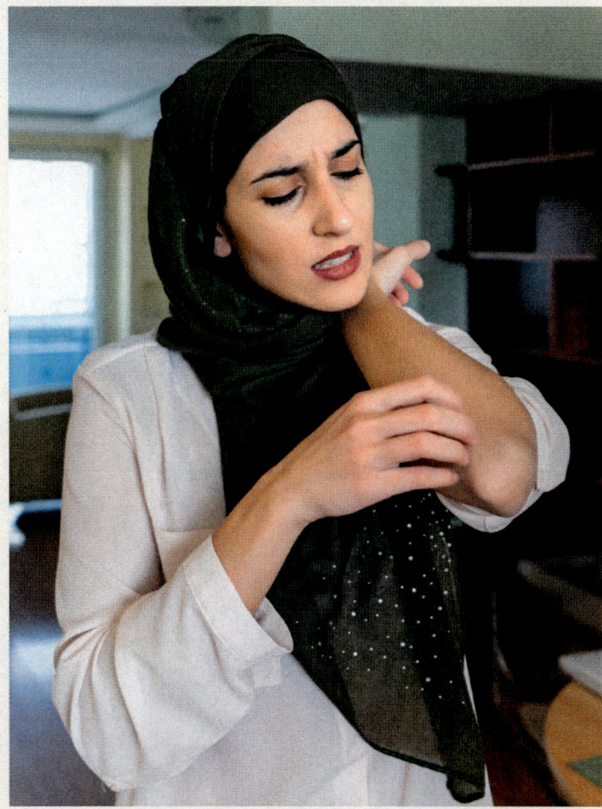

Itch is pain's more poorly understood cousin. The two share some neural pathways, but not all.

Hijacking The Brain

New research suggests that the brain's reward system has different mechanisms for craving and pleasure. Craving is driven by the neurotransmitter dopamine. Pleasure is stimulated by other neurotransmitters in "hedonic hot spots." When the craving circuitry overwhelms the pleasure hot spots, addiction occurs, leading people to pursue a behavior or drug despite the consequences.

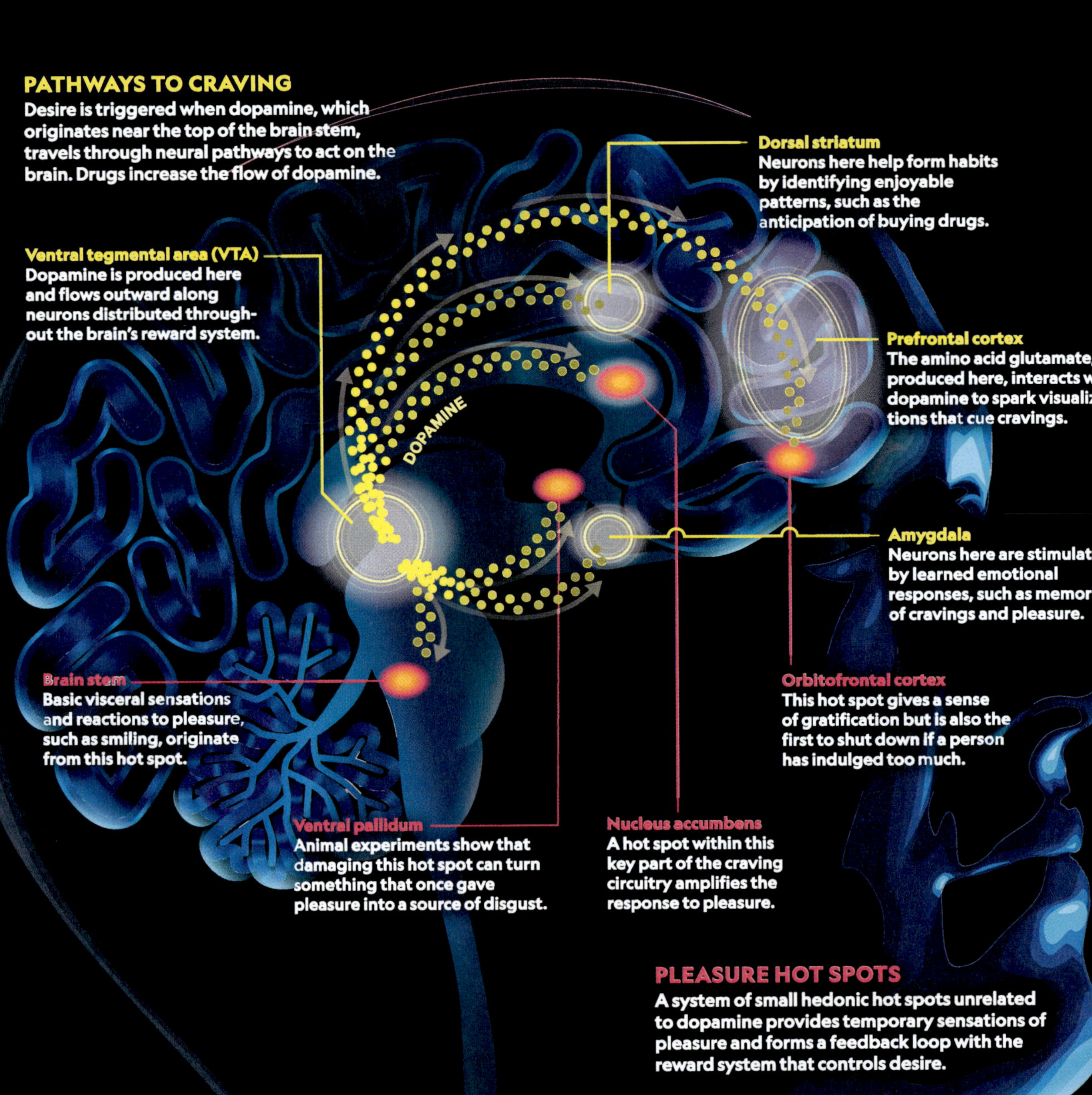

NEURON ACTIVITY

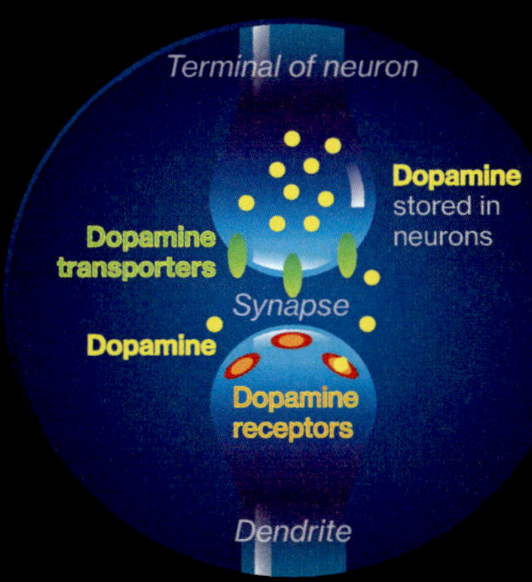

In a normal state
Neurotransmitters carry nerve impulses across synapses between cells to excite or inhibit activity.

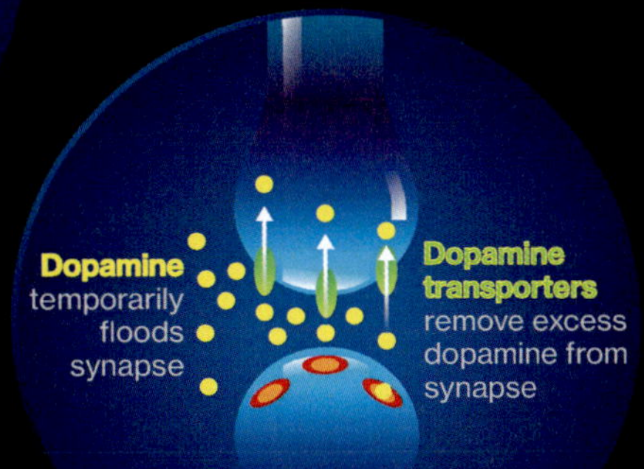

In an excited state
Dopamine temporarily floods a synapse when a pleasurable activity, such as gambling, sex, shopping, or gaming, is anticipated or experienced.

A NATURAL HIGH

Our brains evolved a dopamine-based reward system to encourage behaviors that help us survive, such as eating, procreating, and interacting socially.

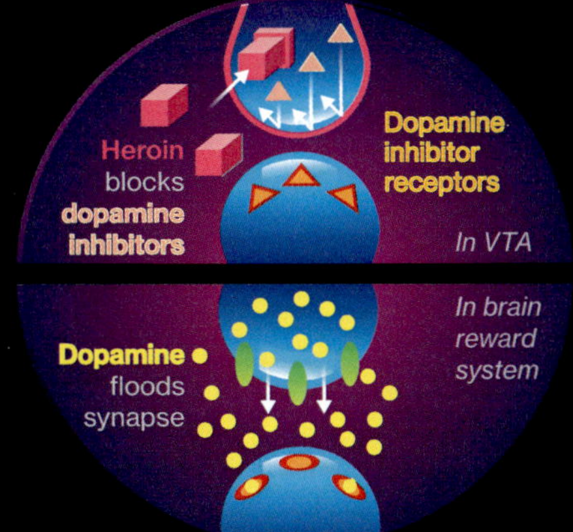

On heroin
Synapses flood with dopamine when heroin blocks dopamine inhibitors in the VTA.

A CHEMICAL RUSH

Different drugs interact with the reward system in unique ways to keep synapses artificially flooded with dopamine. This dopamine rush can rewire your brain to want more drugs, leading to addiction.

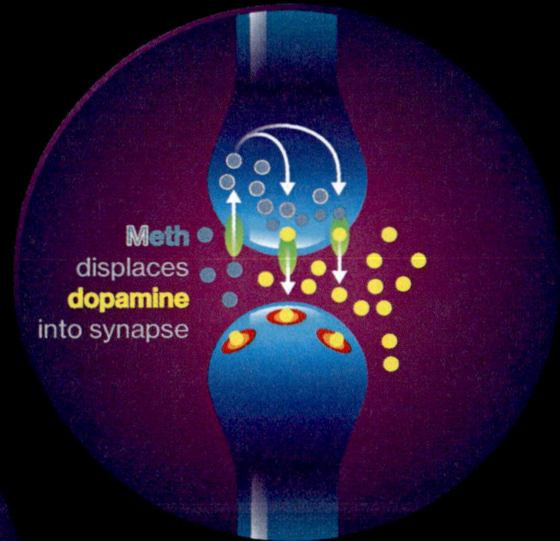

On methamphetamine
The drug reverses the natural, controlled flow of dopamine into neurons, forcing dopamine to rush into synapses instead.

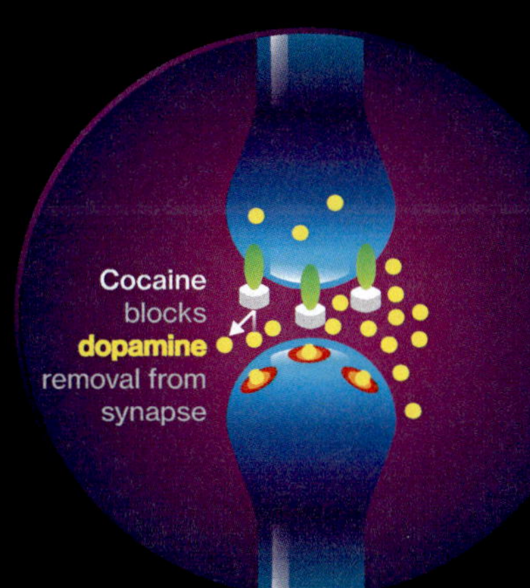

On cocaine
By interfering with dopamine transport, cocaine prevents the removal of excess dopamine from synapses.

JASON TREAT AND RYAN T. WILLIAMS, NGM STAFF
ART: DANIEL HERTZBERG
SOURCE: KENT BERRIDGE, UNIVERSITY OF MICHIGAN

of play—and instead has everything to do with the basic body-colliding elements the game requires of its participants. This also makes CTE a you-and-me problem, not just one for professional athletes.

McKee says one of the most disturbing studies she has worked on was in 2019, when her lab reported that for every 2.6 years of football played at *any* level—high school, college, or professional—an athlete's risk of CTE doubles. The culprit is the types of hits to the head that are so endemic to the game, and so seemingly mild, that most people play right through them.

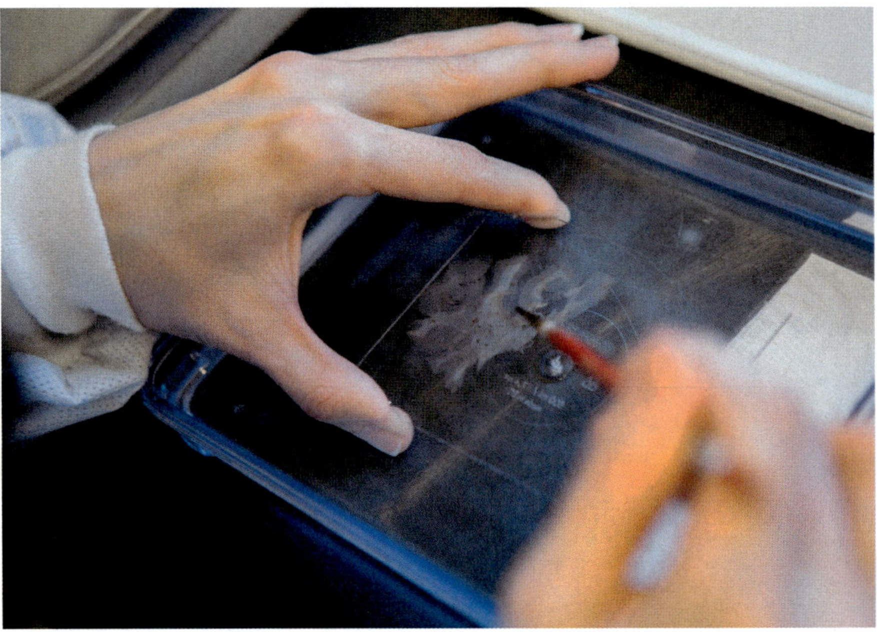

A researcher mounts a brain section on a slide at the brain bank Ann McKee runs.

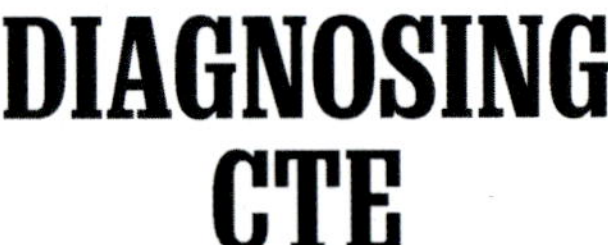

DIAGNOSING CTE

ONE OF THE most frustrating aspects of the human body is that a vital organ carrying your whole life inside its folds is housed in the worst possible place: inside a skull bone rife with sharp protrusions just waiting to poke the brain's delicate tissue. Every time an impact hits the body, this perilous design shows its faults. It's like shaking a ripe raspberry inside a walnut shell. "I don't think we're making a dent at all in really how many players right now are at risk for CTE," McKee says. And the public's focus on sports overshadows how the same reality affects those experiencing repeated head trauma from domestic violence, uncontrolled seizures, or military service.

> **For every 2.6 years of football played at *any* level—high school, college, or professional—an athlete's risk of CTE doubles.**

Like climate scientists, she feels she's "talking into the void. What will it take for people to wake up?"

Probably something shocking, like a way of identifying CTE in the living, not just the deceased. Finding biomarkers of the disease in blood or cerebrospinal fluid—the liquid that surrounds the brain and spinal cord—is key to that advance. McKee thinks that's about five years away, which would be 23 years since she unknowingly encountered her first brain with the disease.

In 2003, she was toiling away inspecting postmortem brain tissue from people who had Alzheimer's disease, looking for something that would explain what makes one person age healthfully and another not so much. She was obsessed with tau, the misbehaving class of proteins that Alzheimer's and CTE broadly have in common, although different types of tau underlie each disease.

McKee came in on weekends to do extremely finicky, microscopic work, updating enormous spreadsheets full of data as she went. "I felt that if I just paid enough attention to one particular issue, I would discover something that no one else had seen before," McKee recalls. And then she did, but it wasn't what she expected.

While poring over brain tissue from a 72-year-old who, 15 years earlier, had been diagnosed with a supposed case of Alzheimer's, she saw a pattern of tau proteins that looked nothing like the tangles characteristic of Alzheimer's.

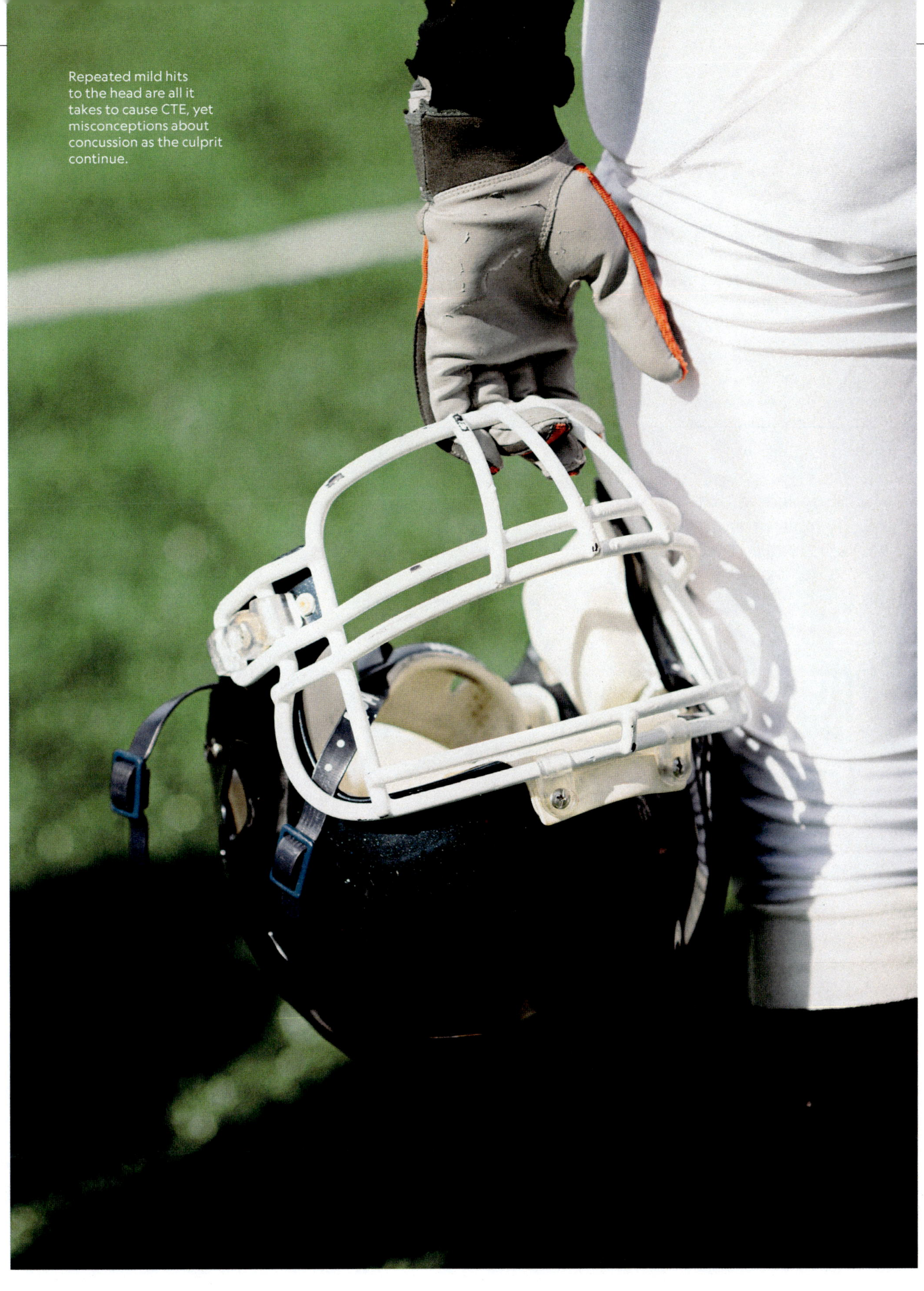

Repeated mild hits to the head are all it takes to cause CTE, yet misconceptions about concussion as the culprit continue.

After the autopsy, McKee learned the man whose brain she had examined had been a world champion boxer.

"I'd seen hundreds and hundreds of brains by then, but when I saw the boxer's brain . . . , " she says, then pauses. She's told her origin story so many times—including when the *Boston Globe* named her Bostonian of the Year in 2017, and when she was on *Time*'s list of the 100 Most Influential People in 2018—but this flash in her personal history still catches her. Finally, she laughs incredulously, and tries again to put the pivotal moment into words: "It's just . . . I'd never seen anything like it. It was like, 'Holy Christmas, what is this?'"

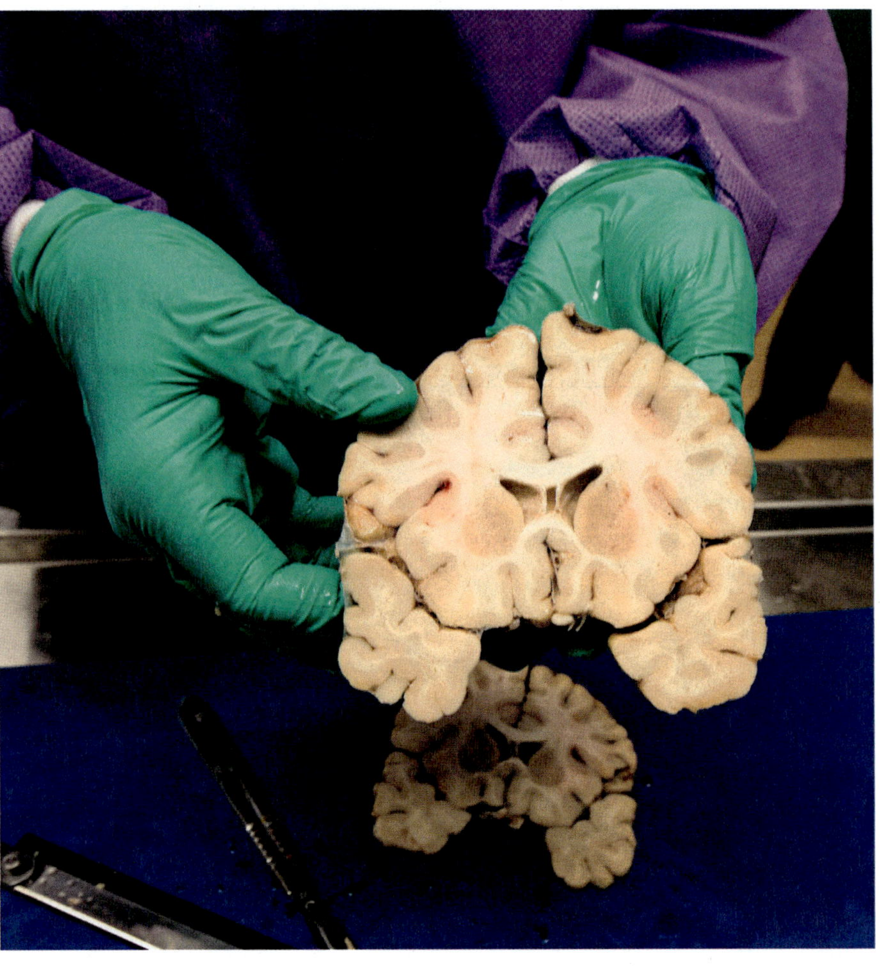

Many NFL players who die young, of supposed CTE, donate their brains to Ann McKee's research. Here, she autopsies a brain from a player in his 40s.

FOR THE LOVE OF BRAINS

THERE WAS A long stretch between the boxer brain and the accolades during which McKee's work fell prey to intra-neuroscience criticism. She wasn't publishing enough academic papers, her peers said. And she leaned too heavily on pictures—where were her graphs? Without this specific kind of scientific rigor, others perceived her to be in a quagmire of confirmation bias, only seeing what she wanted to see in the patterns of someone else's brain tissue. McKee's findings about CTE were simply too observational, naysayers concluded.

"That's scientific discovery for me, I'm a neuropathologist," she says now, still bristling. "It's like, 'I know *you* can't see this under the microscope, but I can, and this is what I do.' This is what I spent my whole life doing. To me it was black and white."

SHE LIKENS HER process to Darwin or Galileo—the foundation of robust science, to her, is in first noticing patterns in the world around you that are invisible to everyone else. Later, the walls are built of data. "A lot of [science] starts with keen, astute observation, and paying attention," she says.

But McKee played ball with the criticism, so to speak (not football, of course; the born and raised Green Bay Packers Cheesehead cut that out of her entertainment diet years ago when the reality of her discoveries began to sink in). She founded the brain bank, which today houses about 1,200 brains. She collected data, she made those graphs—and enlarged pictures of microscope slides to a scale where even an untrained eye could appreciate a pattern lifting from the noise. She published hundreds of papers. And in 2011 she testified before the U.S. Congress about the prevalence of CTE in athletes and military members. "Now . . . we're flooded with data, and everything that we originally hypothesized actually was confirmed," she laughs.

McKee still has many questions about how this disease works. Although tau is key to diagnosing CTE posthumously, there's still no clear link between the protein and the most devastating aspect of the disease: the personality changes that can destroy a person's life and sense of self and lead them to take their own life. "So what is it in the brain that makes those changes?" she wonders. "That's actually one of the most critical questions." About 150 of the brains she has access to right now are from donors under the age of 34; a majority died by suicide.

THERE IS ALSO a paucity of women's brains in the bank McKee runs, leaving open many questions about whether the risks of CTE have any differences across the sexes, an increasing concern as professional women's sports gain more traction and more women sign up for military service. There is also, of course, the perennial nature-versus-nurture question: How much of this neurodegenerative response to brain injury is genetic, and how much of it is because of specific life events?

But in the end, it's not the promise of going down any one of these pathways of scientific inquiry that keeps McKee coming back day after day, it's just a pure love of brains. "There's just so many mysteries about the brain that I can be very passionate about doing brain science," she says. "To me, it defines us."

As Ann McKee has toiled away researching the risks of CTE, there has been tremendous resistance to the societal change her findings seem to urge.

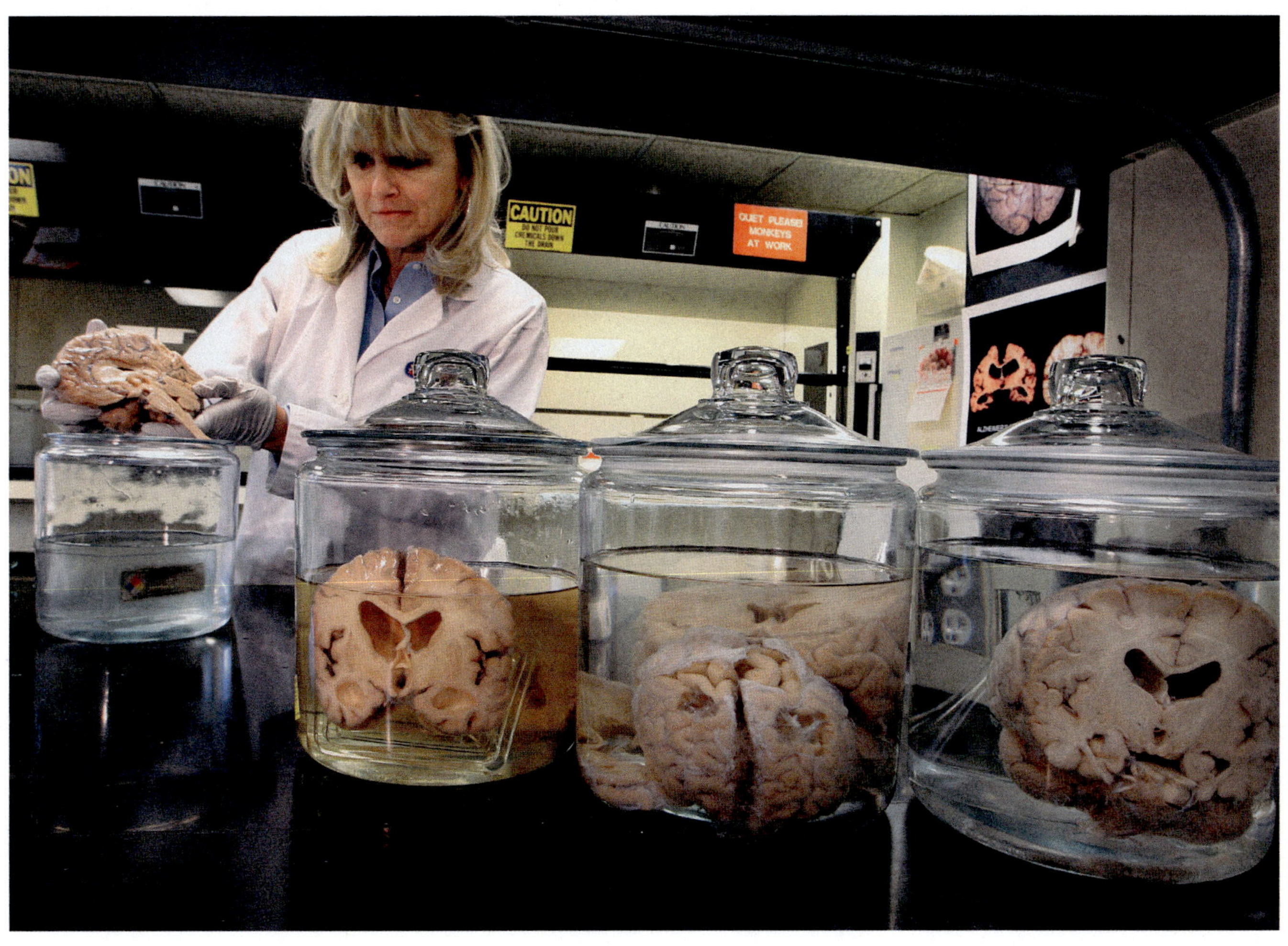

CHAPTER 4

THE "EASY" PROBLEMS OF CONSCIOUSNESS

Chipping away at the mysteries of coma, sleep, psychedelic drugs, and anesthesia can explain how consciousness works, although we may never know why we have it.

Athena Demertzi may be a neuroscientist who studies human consciousness, but she tries not to think too hard about it. "I end up dealing with existential issues and daily problems," she says. The focus for her is not: Why do we have consciousness? Instead, it's the secondary question: Why does consciousness work in some people's brains, but not in the brains of others?

For centuries, the job of answering the first question fell to philosophers and religious leaders. When the study of brain physiology began to emerge as a discipline in the mid-1800s, scientists ignored consciousness, viewing human self-awareness as a given, unbefitting scientific exploration and explanation. But to a contemporary generation of neuroscientists, even if you can never answer the colossal question of why we have consciousness, trying to explain how it functions is essential.

Drawing a clear picture of how the brain maintains consciousness, or drifts in and out of different levels of consciousness, is key to creating treatments for those who lose it unexpectedly as well as better managing the medication used to make surgery bearable. Consciousness is the most astonishing act our big, complex, interconnected brains pull off when they're working properly, and scientists are only just beginning to understand it.

For centuries, understanding human consciousness was relegated to religion and philosophy, and not a line of inquiry the natural sciences would tackle. Now, however, with increasingly sophisticated technology at our fingertips, it's considered the final frontier of neuroscience.

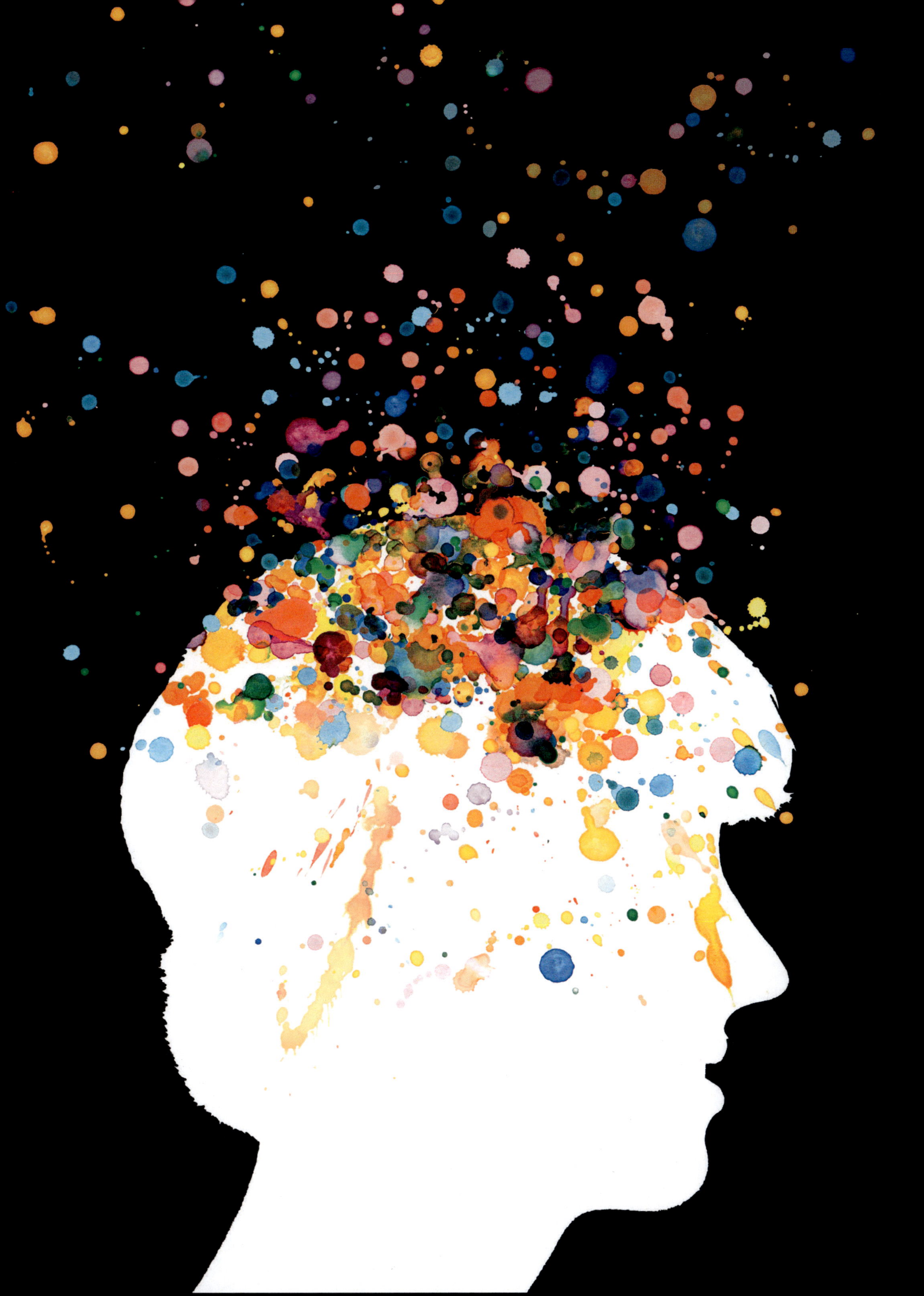

THE PROBLEMS OF CONSCIOUSNESS

HOW DOES ONE begin to crack a nut as big as consciousness? By breaking it first in half, and slowly working to further pick apart one side. Consciousness studies can be loosely divided into two realms: the hard and easy problems.

"The hard problem is, where does . . . my inner experience come from?" says Albert Garcia-Romeu, an assistant professor at the Johns Hopkins Center for Psychedelic and Consciousness Research. In other words: What is the origin of consciousness, and where is it located in the brain? French philosopher René Descartes tried to answer this question in 1637. He hypothesized in his posthumously published book *Treatise of Man* that the pineal gland was the site of the human soul and all its inner thoughts (we now know it secretes melatonin and helps modulate sleep states). "Unfortunately, I don't think [consciousness] can really be localized," says Garcia-Romeu, a stance that defines today's inquiries into this human experience.

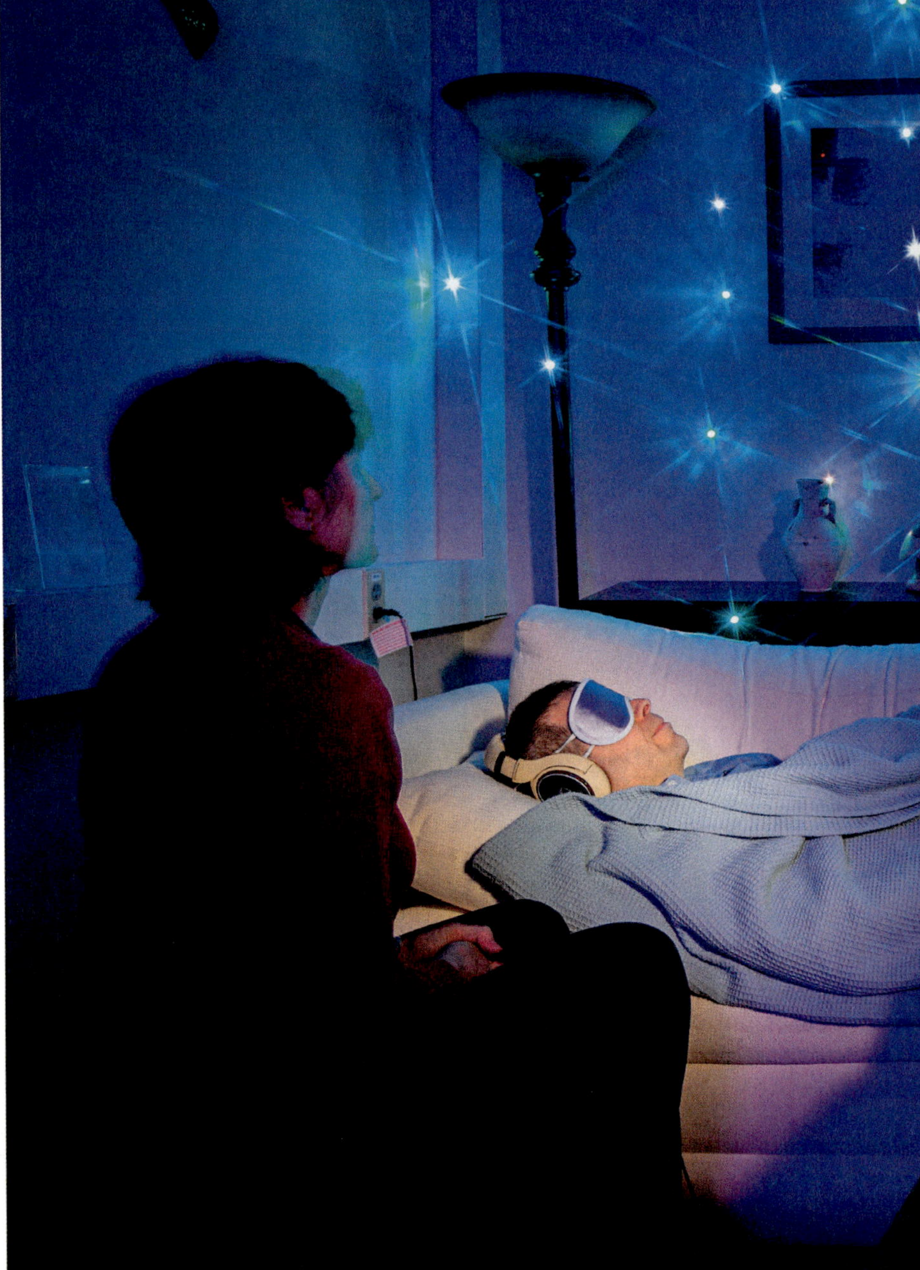

SCIENTISTS NOW TINKER with the "easy" problems of consciousness—which are still quite hard. Consciousness is understood through this lens not as having a locus in the brain or elsewhere, but as being the product of many active neuronal networks communicating in tandem, and giving rise to both internal self-awareness and awareness of the external environment.

The Glasgow Coma Scale has long been a standard bedside tool for assessing a person's responsiveness to their environment, and is used as a proxy for measuring consciousness in critical health care situations. The behavioral test takes about two minutes to administer and includes tasks such as shining a light into a patient's pupil and looking for dilation, and administering a painful stimulus and looking for a flee response. But using this crude assessment, 42 percent of people diagnosed with unresponsive wakefulness syndrome (formerly called "vegetative state") "actually have some level of

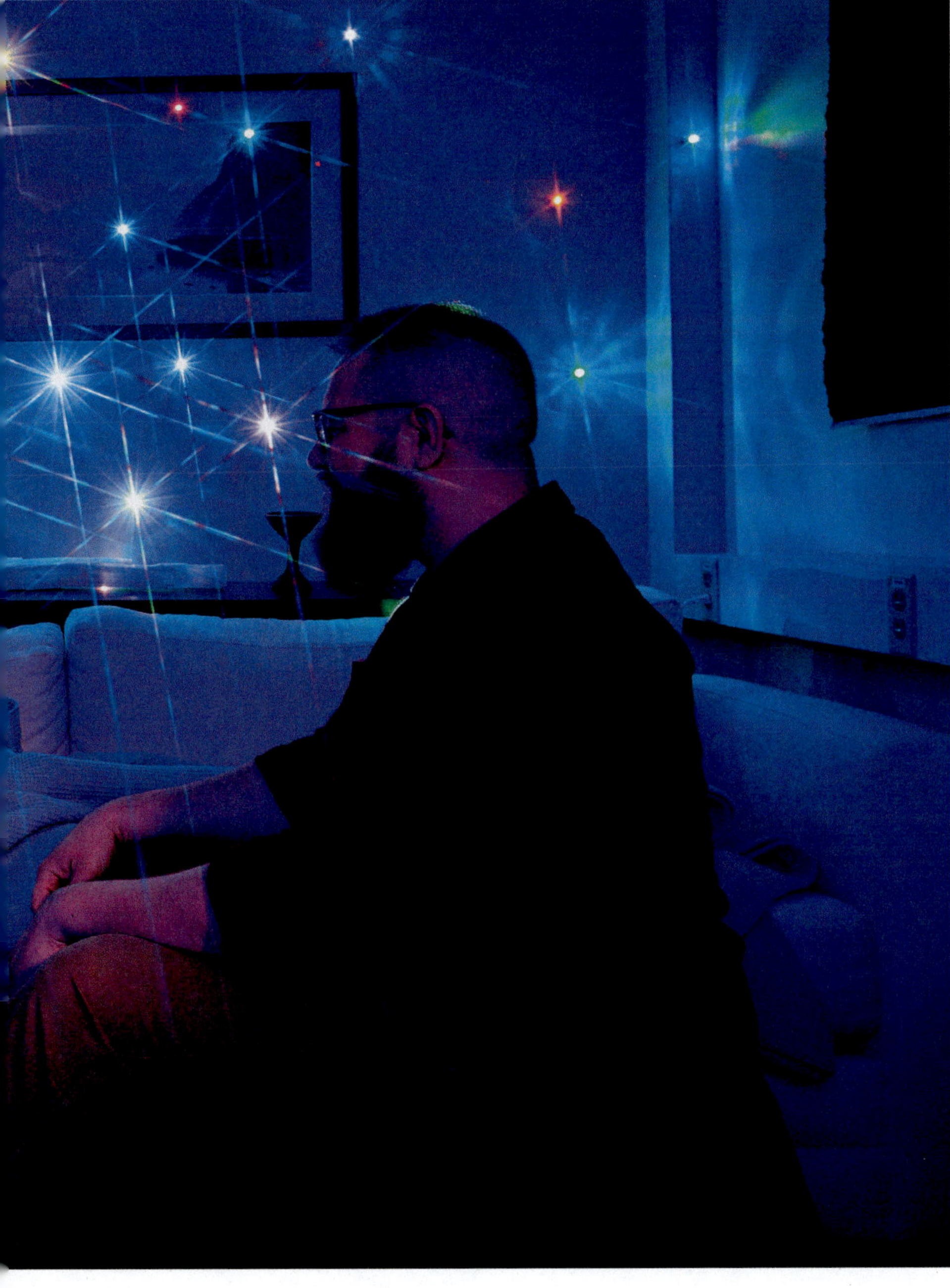

Albert Garcia-Romeu studies how psychedelic drugs, and their consciousness-altering effects, work. Here he is shown in a reenactment of a session to treat addiction.

awareness of themselves or their environment," says Stefanie Blain-Moraes who runs the Biosignal Interaction and Personhood Technology Lab at McGill University in Montreal, Canada.

A POWERFUL TOOL for capturing more nuanced indicators of consciousness is fMRI. The machine measures brain activity by proxy, noting increased levels of blood oxygen in active brain regions. The classic reference point for this application of fMRI is Adrian Owens' 2006 study in *Science*, describing the unexpected brain activity of someone who had been declared unaware of herself and the environment—totally unconscious. When the researchers asked the seemingly unresponsive patient to imagine playing tennis, or picture moving around her house, areas of the brain associated with these activities became active, as though she were really doing them—consistent with how a healthy person's brain would react. "This was the first evidence of covert consciousness," Blain-Moraes says. "The consciousness that could exist in absence of any sort of behavioral responsiveness."

But fMRI isn't used clinically. Intensive care units, where such patients often end up, lack the people power and funding to run such labor intensive and expensive tests. In the ICUs where Blain-Moraes has worked throughout her career, the Glasgow Coma Scale is still the go-to "quick and dirty" diagnostic tool, something that doesn't sit well with those who know there's a more rigorous way out of these woods.

Forty-two percent of people diagnosed with unresponsive wakefulness syndrome (formerly called "vegetative state") actually have some level of awareness.

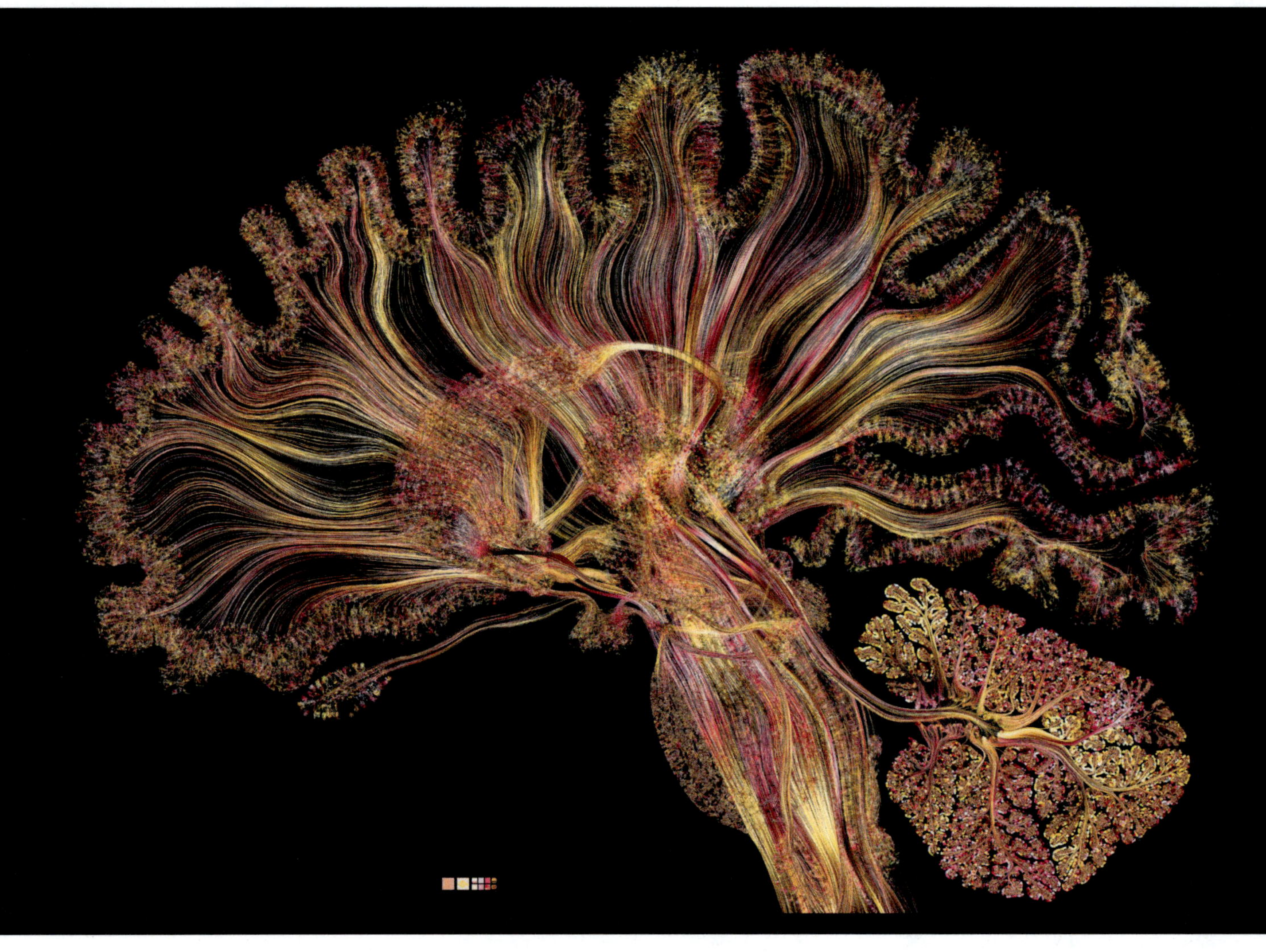

In the micro-etching "Self Reflected in Sunburst," artist-scientists Greg Dunn and Brian Edwards depict their vision of a brain contemplating consciousness—the brain as it perceives itself.

BEFORE EVEN GETTING to the diagnosis point, defining what states of consciousness a person can be in is also complex and debatable. To get a general sense, Blain-Moraes suggests envisioning a graph on which wakefulness is on one axis and awareness is on another. In the bottom left corner of the graph—where wakefulness and awareness are at their lowest—would be something like coma and general anesthesia. Progressing upward along the diagonal line are such milestones as deep sleep, drowsiness, and eventually full wakefulness and awareness. Off the diagonal line are disorders of consciousness, such as intraoperative awareness. This traumatic event occurs when a person is under anesthesia and in a state of medically induced paralysis, but becomes fully aware of their surgery without any external signs they're awake. These are all ways of naming the *level* of someone's consciousness, but there's another element at play that's more about the *contents* of consciousness—what being alive feels like. Some sleep states, such as REM, combine both elements: you can have internal, subjective experiences in the form of dreams while being "unawake" and unaware of your actual external environment. A seizure, for example, may only modulate a person's level of consciousness, while psychedelic drugs may alter just the contents.

FAR OUT

ALBERT GARCIA-ROMEU IS a skeptic. He studies psychedelic drugs, well known to alter consciousness, but he believes they will take us only so far, scientifically, in tackling the hard problem of consciousness—the question of where our sense of self comes from. The drugs can, however, gain us some headway in understanding the many easy problems, such as what underlies emotional experiences.

Users of LSD typically have increased emotional empathy, something that scientists thought resulted from the drug binding to receptors in the brain where the neurotransmitter serotonin usually latches. LSD would then alter communication between neurons, in lieu of the neurotransmitter doing this job. But a 2021 study showed that even when researchers blocked the brain's serotonin receptors, users of LSD still experienced some increased empathy beyond their baseline. The change in emotional state was coming through some additional mechanism. One theory of consciousness is that it's not a singular brain activity with one underlying mechanism, but rather a network of linked behaviors taking place throughout the brain.

Garcia-Romeu eschews the term "hallucinogens" because it can mislead people about what these drugs actually do, and it can also muddy the research around them, which is more about changes in perception than deep consciousness.

"When the Self boundary—or the ego, if you want to call it that—breaks down or dissolves, the understanding of reality and the universe around us is also quite altered," Garcia-Romeu says. "That's sort of where I think the consciousness-altering piece comes in with these drugs." To better learn how deep consciousness works, scientists turn to the type of drug used for anesthesia.

To test psilocybin—colloquially known as mushrooms—as an addiction treatment, Garcia-Romeu administers gelatin capsules, some of which are placebos, in controlled research trials.

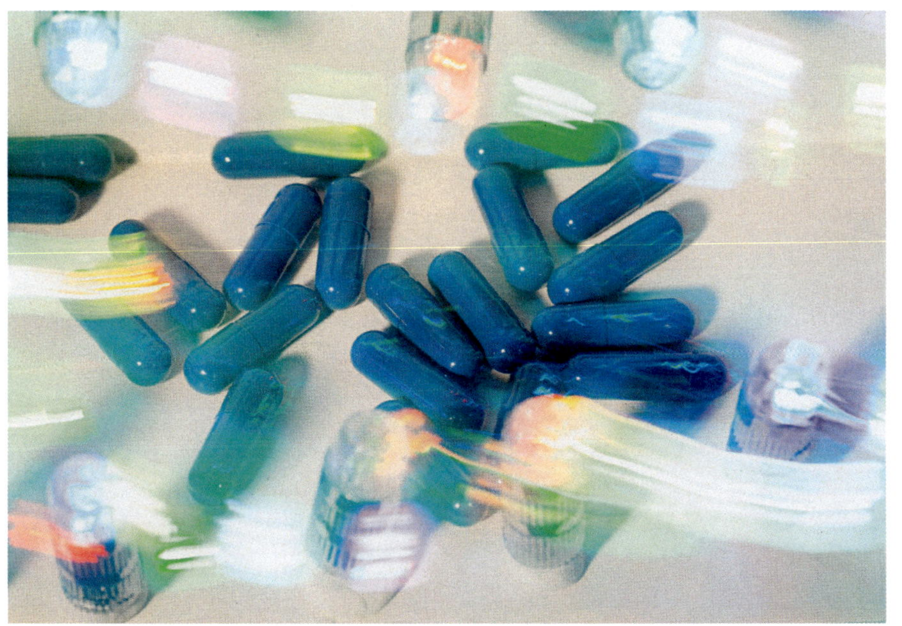

GOING UNDER

DEEP INSIDE MASSACHUSETTS General Hospital is an auspicious, domed room. The convex ceiling is a heavenly sky blue; a window pierces it and fills the space with diffuse sunlight, even on a cloudy day. The half circle of upholstered risers running along the wall make for a calm, contemplative place to sit inside the thrum of one of the busiest hospitals in the world. But about 175 years ago, the room was full of spectators, here to witness the first public demonstration of ether, a chemical used in anesthesia that's fallen out of fashion.

An oil painting framed in gold shows the inaugural, unconscious patient, propped up and bleeding from a dental procedure, as white men in black suits huddle around him, peering and pointing. Now called the Ether Dome, this space is mostly a fancy hallway. And since that demonstration on October 16, 1846, doctors and dentists have used various forms of anesthesia—first ether, nitrous oxide, or chloroform; now propofol, ketamine, or sevoflurane—to reduce patient suffering. They've done so with remarkable safety and precision, considering that for most of that time they had little understanding of how these drugs interact with

Anatomy of Empathy

Using scanning technology, scientists can identify parts of the brain that are active when we empathize with others. By combining these results with other findings—from psychological evaluations to genetic testing—researchers are beginning to determine which biological and environmental factors reinforce or corrode our capacity for empathy.

The Empathy Circuit

Highlighted areas have distinct roles in how the brain responds to others.

- **Viscerally reacting to others' physical pain**
- **Mirroring people's actions and emotions**
- **Reading the eye expressions and movements of others**
- **Imagining thoughts of others** (right side only)

THE AMYGDALA
Extremely altruistic people have more neural activity in their enlarged amygdala—a part of the brain associated with learned emotional responses and the processing of distressing stimuli.

How the circuit is activated

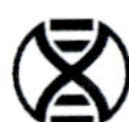

Biological
Genetic variations enable some people to recognize facial expressions better or produce more of an enzyme related to lower aggressiveness.

Psychological
A nurturing childhood can potentially transform someone who is genetically predisposed to lack empathy into a social, nonviolent citizen.

Social
Watching a friend cry or hearing a dog whimper, for example, can evoke empathy and a desire to end what is perceived as shared suffering.

The Empathy Spectrum

Empathy can be measured through empathy quotient (EQ) tests. Questions aim to determine the magnitude of one's interest in how others feel and think. Extreme altruists fall at one end of the spectrum; those who totally lack empathy at the other.

Extreme altruists
Highly empathic people, such as those who risk their lives for strangers, are better able to recognize pain or fear in others' faces.

Professionals in the humanities
People such as musicians and historians typically score higher on EQ tests.

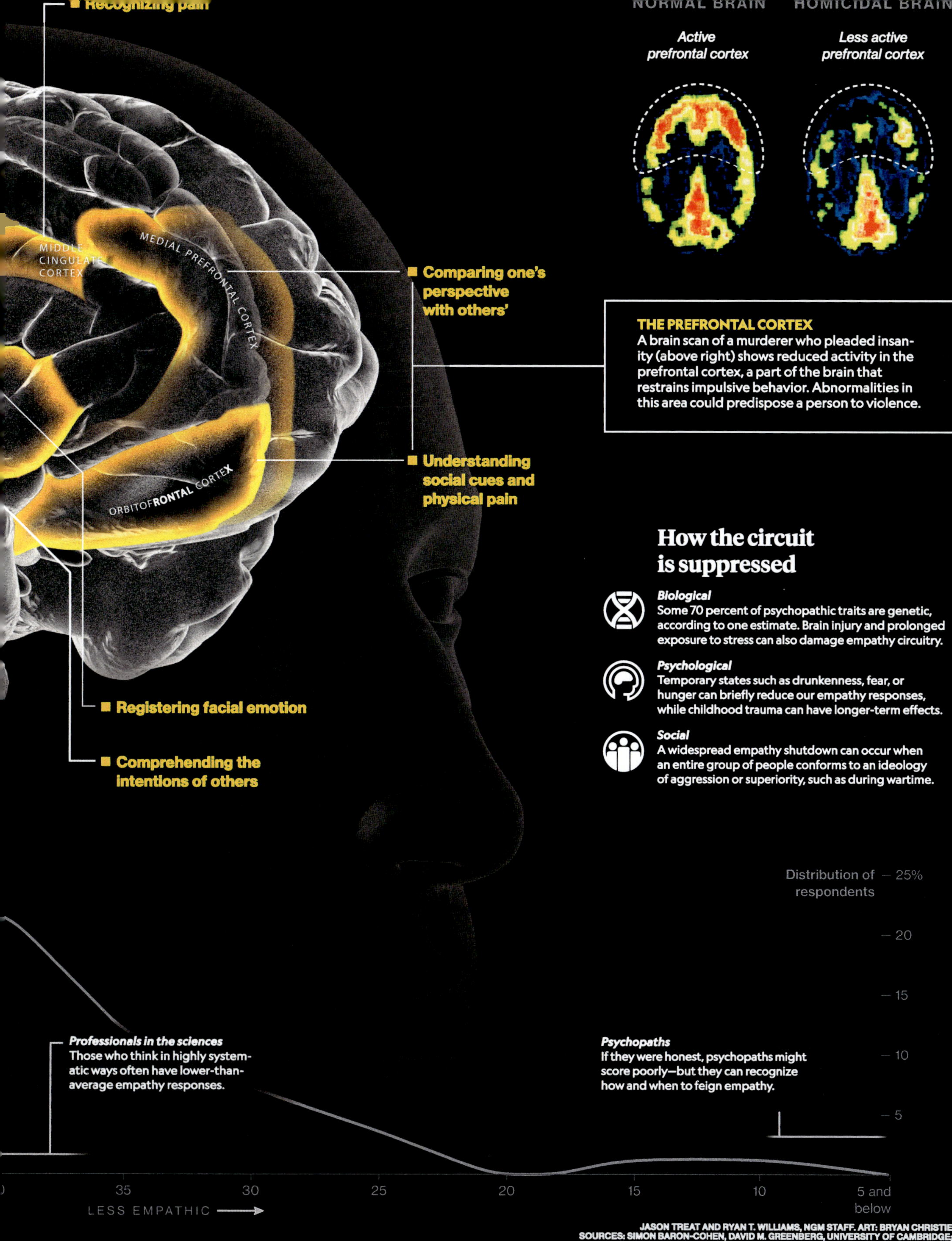

Recognizing pain
MIDDLE CINGULATE CORTEX
MEDIAL PREFRONTAL CORTEX
ORBITOFRONTAL CORTEX
Comparing one's perspective with others'
Understanding social cues and physical pain
Registering facial emotion
Comprehending the intentions of others
NORMAL BRAIN
HOMICIDAL BRAIN
Active prefrontal cortex
Less active prefrontal cortex
THE PREFRONTAL CORTEX
A brain scan of a murderer who pleaded insanity (above right) shows reduced activity in the prefrontal cortex, a part of the brain that restrains impulsive behavior. Abnormalities in this area could predispose a person to violence.
How the circuit is suppressed
Biological
Some 70 percent of psychopathic traits are genetic, according to one estimate. Brain injury and prolonged exposure to stress can also damage empathy circuitry.
Psychological
Temporary states such as drunkenness, fear, or hunger can briefly reduce our empathy responses, while childhood trauma can have longer-term effects.
Social
A widespread empathy shutdown can occur when an entire group of people conforms to an ideology of aggression or superiority, such as during wartime.
Distribution of respondents
25%
20
15
10
5
Professionals in the sciences
Those who think in highly systematic ways often have lower-than-average empathy responses.
Psychopaths
If they were honest, psychopaths might score poorly—but they can recognize how and when to feign empathy.
35
30
25
20
15
10
5 and below
LESS EMPATHIC
JASON TREAT AND RYAN T. WILLIAMS, NGM STAFF. ART: BRYAN CHRISTIE
SOURCES: SIMON BARON-COHEN, DAVID M. GREENBERG, UNIVERSITY OF CAMBRIDGE;

the brain. And until recently, what scientists knew about how anesthesia progressively turns off consciousness vastly outpaced what they knew about how the brain turns consciousness back on when anesthesia lifts.

ABOUT 15 YEARS ago, scientists discovered that the process of losing consciousness works like this: An anesthesiologist administers a drug, the drug binds to receptors in the brain, and a state of controlled unconsciousness sets in, starting with the prefrontal cortex and moving into the parietal cortex. They assumed that when the anesthesiologist stopped drug flow, the molecules became unbound from those receptors in the brain and processes or activities that were suppressed came back to life in the reverse order in which they turned off. That is, the parietal cortex would come back online first, followed by the prefrontal cortex. "Then it became clear that's actually not the case," says George Mashour, chair of anesthesiology at Michigan Medicine, the University of

"The First Operation With Ether," painted by Robert Cutler Hinckley in 1882, commemorates the first public demonstration of anesthesia in 1846 and is displayed in an amphitheater now known as the Ether Dome at Massachusetts General Hospital.

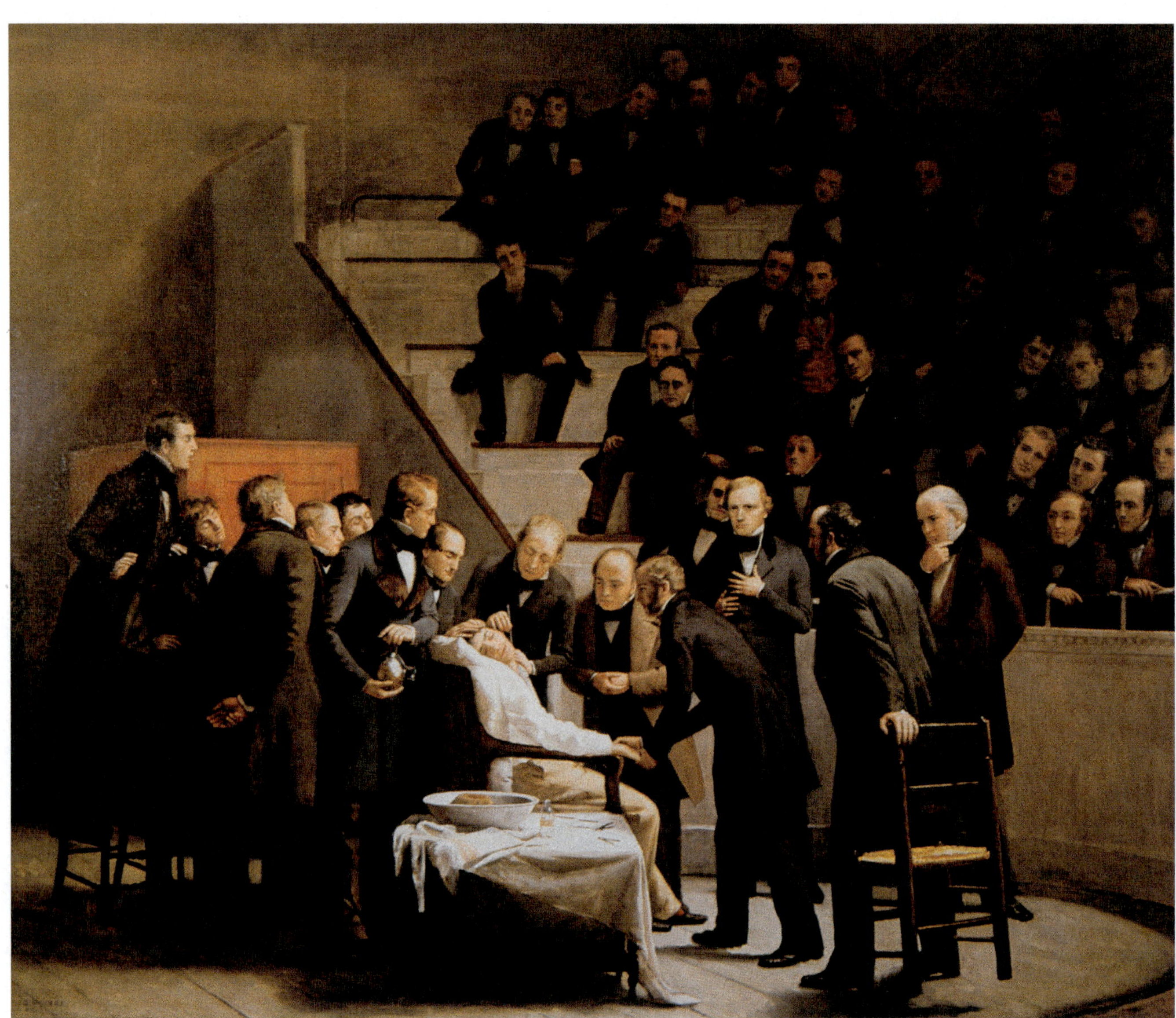

STAYING AWAKE FOR BRAIN SURGERY

During most major surgeries, patients lie blessedly unconscious. But not during brain surgery—a surgery you might instinctively most want to be *un*aware of. The brain is a precarious arrangement of tissue, blood vessels, and cells all stuffed into a relatively small area: 233 to 465 square inches (1,500 to 3,000 sq cm) of tissue folded neatly into the skull. One infinitesimal mistake in touching this organ, and you could impair someone for life. That's why brain surgeons do part of their work while a patient is awake—physically numb to the pain and emotionally numb to the anxiety, but responsive.

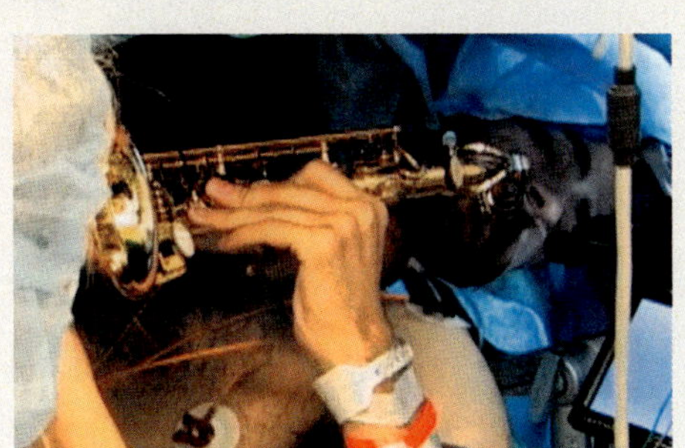

Using electrodes to stimulate different regions of the brain, surgeons can work out a map of the patient's brain, a kind of guide for how far to travel and where to stop once surgical tools and potential damage are involved. They need the patient's feedback for this. "Does this make your tongue tingle?" they might ask while placing one electrode, or, "Can you tell me your name?" while they place another.

Accessing a live brain is so extreme that it's not something neuroscientists get to do very often, instead relying primarily on behavioral tests or brain imaging to get a sense for how this organ works. So, when a health issue brings someone in for surgery, it offers a secondary opportunity to learn more about the brain in action up close, not by proxy.

In 2017, researchers at the University of Rochester saw a patient with a tumor in the brain that changed his ability to hear music in stereo. The patient was himself a musician. The primary issue was safely removing the tumor, but the secondary opportunity was to better understand how the brain hears and processes music. The patient (above) played his saxophone during the surgery.

Michigan's academic medical center. Entering and emerging from unconsciousness are "not mirror images, they're distinct neural processes."

In a 2021 study, Mashour gave 30 healthy patients the same type of general anesthesia people normally receive during surgery—although the participants did not undergo any procedures—and then checked their cognitive function in a progressive battery of tests for three hours as they emerged from the anesthesia. He vividly remembers watching the first participant's emergence in shock.

"This young man who had been anesthetized, he woke up so groggy," Mashour recalls. "We're sitting him up, we're helping him get the computer in front of him with the cognitive tests, and then he just starts nailing these abstract matching questions. I've done these tests . . . they were not easy. We were all looking at each other just like, 'Wait a minute, what's going on here?' I thought it might be a fluke, but of course, it ended up panning out rigorously."

Those matching questions test the prefrontal cortex's function, the part of the brain that enables you to make complex plans. But if a person coming off anesthesia can barely stand, why is their high-level prefrontal cortex up and running? Mashour thinks it's an evolutionary advantage that helps us stay safe from predators during sleep, another state of fluctuating consciousness that we can emerge from far more quickly than drug-induced unconsciousness. If you were sleeping, and woke to an intruder breaking into your home, it would be critical to rapidly assess the situation and make

Understanding the neurobiology of how someone emerges from anesthesia can support better patient outcomes after surgery, an hours-long process with some unkind side effects.

decisions about how to stay safe before anything else. The same would've been true for our ancestors, living and sleeping among nature's many threats.

Understanding the neurobiology of how someone emerges from anesthesia can support better patient outcomes after surgery, an hours-long process with some unkind side effects, such as temporary memory deficits and nausea. But this study also cracks open the door to bigger questions, such as: "How does the brain reconstitute consciousness and cognition?" Mashour says. "If we knew that, it might help us better understand . . . pathologic states of unconsciousness, such as coma."

SONG OF THE SELF

ONE OF THESE so-called easy problems of consciousness—which, again, is extremely hard—is finding ways to overcome communication gaps between the conscious and unconscious, or between the conscious and noncommunicative. If a patient who physiologically reacts to the external world in only minute ways is also experiencing their own rich, internal world, but their caregivers have no idea, there's a tremendous risk for suffering on both ends. Creating a tool that builds a bridge between them is paramount and a bit ethically dubious. But mostly it's just very complex. The first step is finding reliable ways to assess a person's level of consciousness.

"I've learned through hard experience that if you build a technology that

Among the many urgent reasons for better understanding human consciousness is to help facilitate communication, and reduce suffering, for the unconscious and their caretakers.

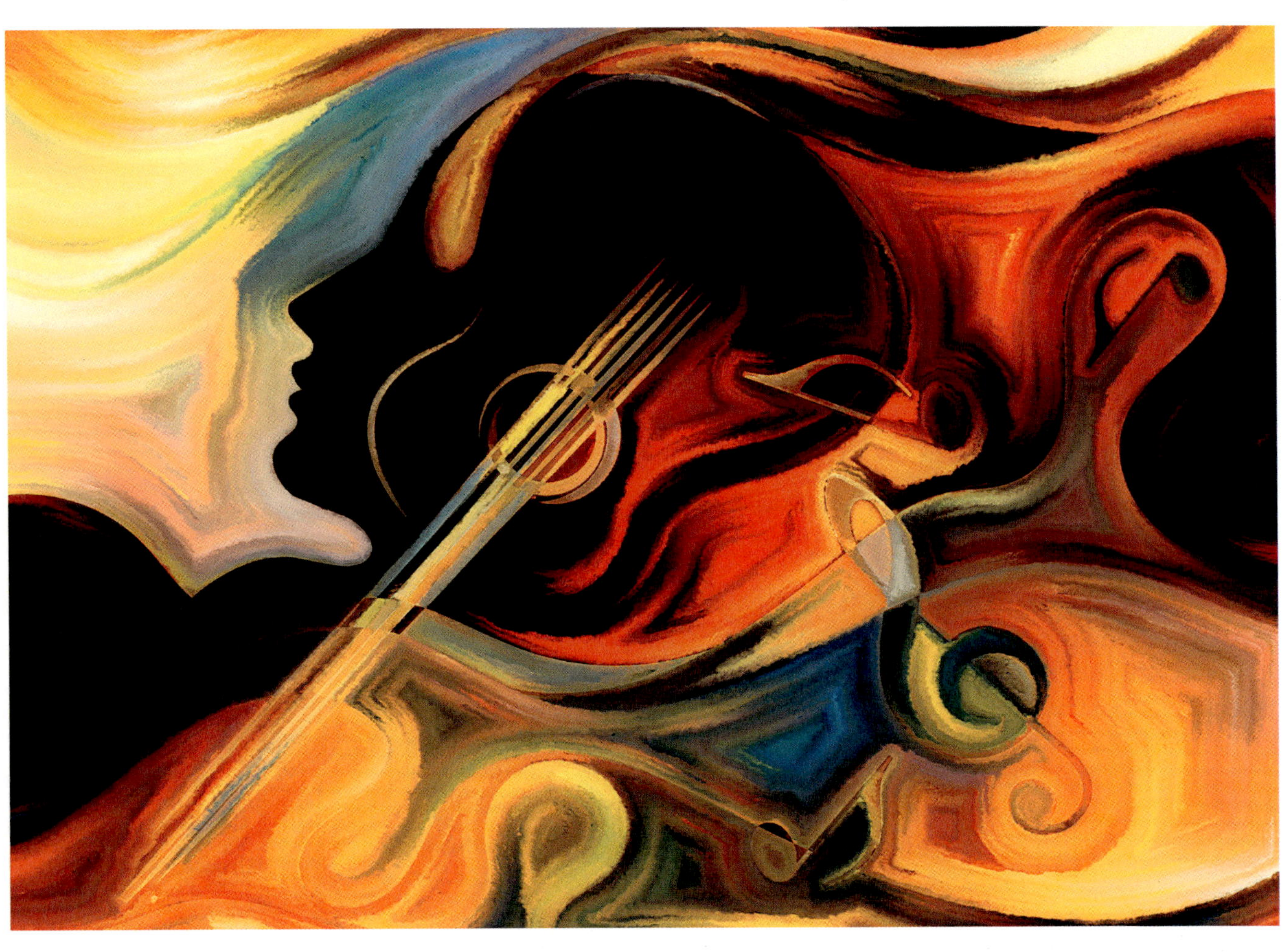

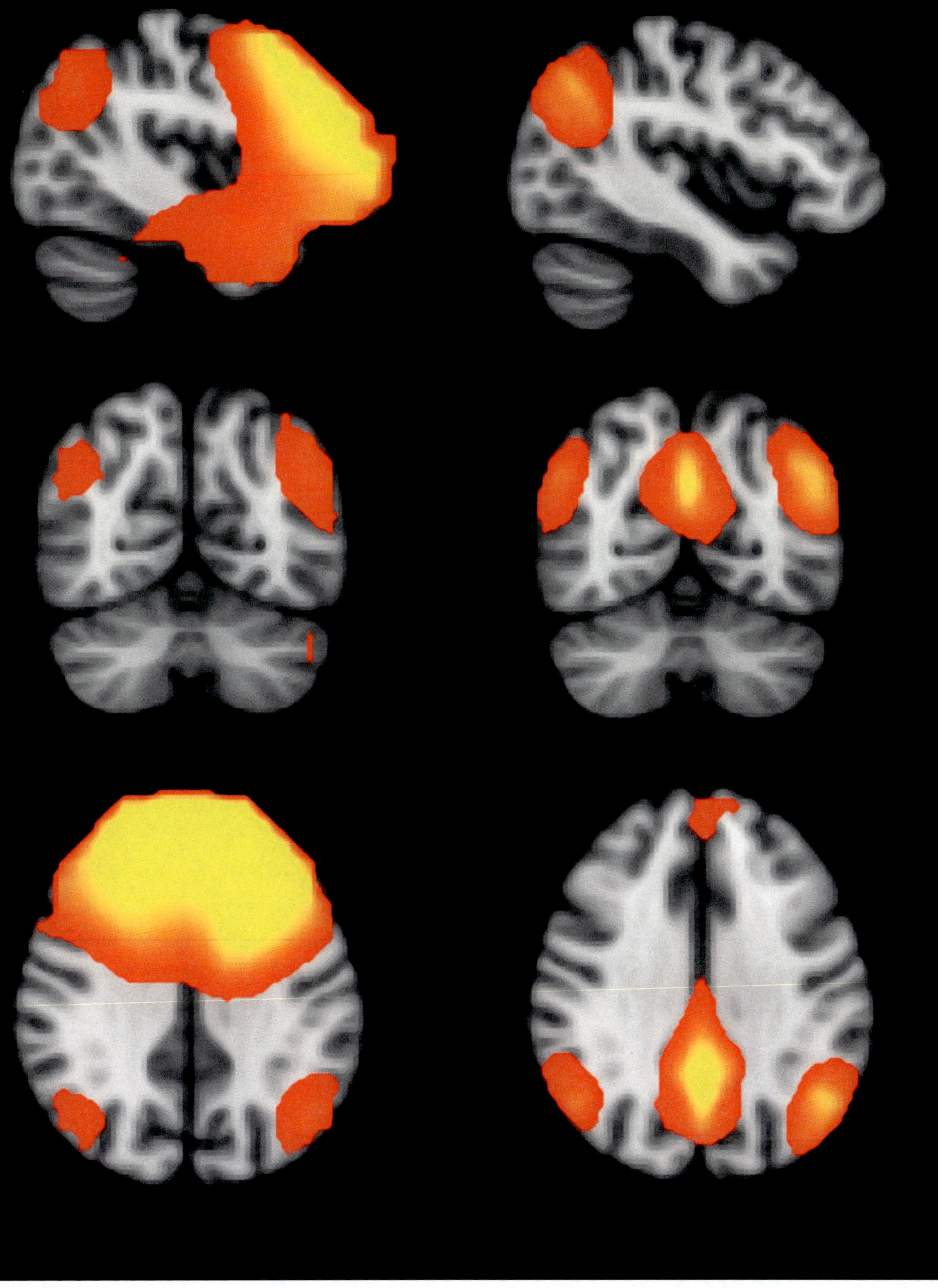

Magnetoencephalography (MEG) scans show activity during the brain's default mode, at rest without undertaking tasks.

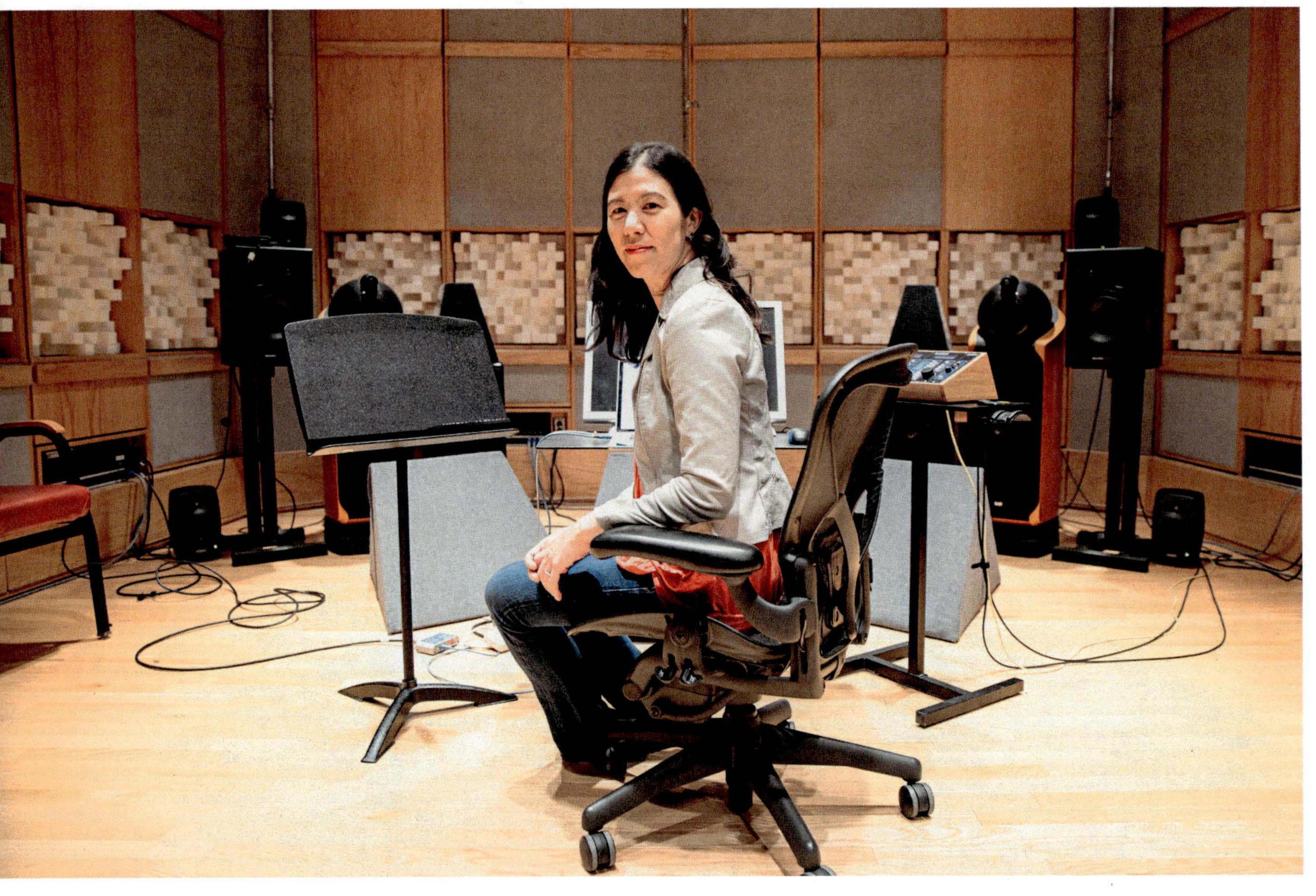

Fusing neuroscience and music, Stefanie Blain-Morales builds tools for those who can't use words to communicate their internal state.

allows you to interact with someone through their physiological signals, and you're not sure that they're conscious, it doesn't work," Blain-Moraes says. "You have to be confident that the other person is aware of you in order to develop some sort of meaningful interaction."

To confidently make this diagnosis, she takes advantage of what she knows about how anesthesia works to turn off consciousness—some of which she learned from Mashour, formerly her postdoctoral fellowship supervisor. First, she assesses a patient's baseline brain activity, then she administers anesthesia and carefully looks for changes. One of the signs she checks for through EEG is the brain's connectivity over a few hours.

In a healthy, conscious person's brain, information in the brain should flow front to back—the frontal lobe is sending information to the parietal lobe where, among other things, the somatosensory cortex lives, which helps you sense the world. Under anesthesia, the informational flow flips and starts moving back to front. Even in the brain of a person suffering major trauma—where entire areas of the brain may have been damaged or removed—information will still move in a reverse order through whatever brain areas are functioning, if there is some level of consciousness. So if this flipped information highway shows up in a test, the next step is figuring out how to measure an unconscious or noncommunicative person's reactive physiology in a way that caregivers can understand.

At first, Blain-Moraes, a biomedical engineer by training, tried doing this in the language she speaks: graphs. The graphs attempted to show many aspects of physiology at once, such as sweat on the skin, temperature in the fingertips, pulse, and blood volume, all of which can be used as various indicators that the brain is mediating some kind of concerted reaction to an external event. Looking at only one aspect would show an incomplete picture—the body doesn't exist in a vacuum—but showing them all together was too much for the average person to visually understand.

Blain-Moraes is not just an engineer, though. She also trained in classical piano at Toronto's Royal Conservatory of Music. And that's how she realized that musicians make holistic sense of parallel streams of information all the time. Musicians can hear the gestalt of all instruments in concert, but they can also key in on simply the bassoon line. Without knowing how to play instruments themselves, lay listeners can still make cognitive sense of the sounds they hear: This movement is slow and feels maudlin; the one before it was rapid and chipper. "I thought, 'Well, there we go—let's use that,'" Blain-Moraes says.

IN 2018, SHE started working on biomusic, a musical communication of a person's physiological states that others could make sense of without using words. While not directly measuring brain activity, it gives another person an immediate sense of the internal experience of someone who can't verbally communicate with them, whether because they're in an unresponsive wakeful state or they're a healthy person with nonverbal autism. There's a customizable aspect to the tool that people with some ability to communicate can use if they wish to express themselves with sounds that aren't music. "We've done work with adolescents with autism who really like trains. When there's . . . a big spike in your skin sweat, you can map that to a woo-woo sound," Blain-Moraes says, mimicking the punctuated horn of a locomotive.

Although biomusic is designed to support caregivers of noncommunicative people, its process raises ethical questions about potentially stripping a person of experiencing the contents of consciousness in privacy. "It's an excellent question," Blain-Moraes says. "Think about what your body does when someone that you love walks into the room . . . If you're an adolescent who hasn't told the person that you like them, do you really want all of that on display?"

HOW TO DONATE A BRAIN

In the United States, there's a fairly smooth pipeline for donating organs: You can sign up to become an organ donor when acquiring a driver's license. Should you die, this simple red heart symbol on your ID will alert the health care system that you've consented to have healthy internal organs, such as a heart or a liver, given over to support someone else's life. But on this long list of donatable organs, one is conspicuously absent: the brain. Donating a brain to scientific discovery is a whole different process, and one that has no centralized form.

Although a brain can't be transplanted, having access to postmortem human brain tissue is an important tool in understanding this vital organ. Only so much work can be done through behavioral tests and digital tools. For those interested in donating their brain to science, one place to start is the National Institute on Aging—part of the National Institutes of Health—which uses them for research on Parkinson's, Huntington's, Alzheimer's, and other diseases.

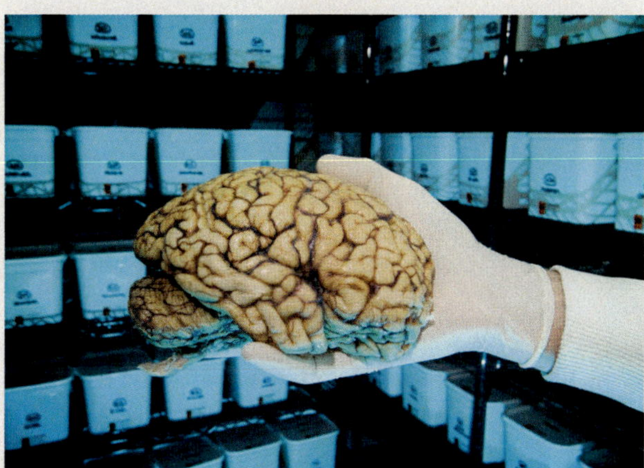

A human brain inside a donation bank

A CLOSER LOOK

ACCESSING THE DEEP BRAIN

A pioneering surgical technique treats a tough form of epilepsy while also giving a rare close-up of the insula, a structure crucial to consciousness and treacherous to access.

Camille LaRock's seizures looked nothing like the ones people see in movies. She stayed fully conscious and could move well enough to play soccer in the midst of a seizure. The only outside sign was a twitch in her eye, a slight droop to her face, and an uncontrollable moan emanating from her lips. The seizures began in middle school, and disrupted life throughout her teens, sometimes multiple times a day. She was on so much anti-seizure medication at one point that she had to lean against the wall to walk between classes. And yet, even with all that medication, the seizures didn't stop.

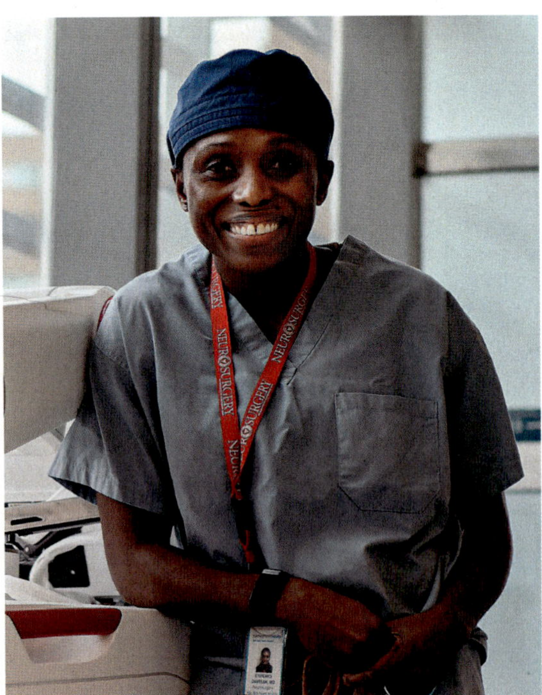

"I felt like I wasn't really living," the 19-year-old says. With nothing to lose, she signed up for an experimental surgery at the hands of Eyiyemisi Damisah, a neurosurgeon at the Yale School of Medicine. When LaRock was 17, Damisah robotically reached deep into her brain to remove a tiny sliver of the insula, an area not commonly seen or accessed.

Exploring the Insula

The insula is "like an island," Damisah says. It helps maintain homeostasis, arousal, and consciousness while hidden beneath critical layers of cortex that orchestrate our big life experiences—memory, language, movement, decision-making. From the body, blood vessels course into the brain, getting smaller, but denser, the deeper they go. For a neurosurgeon entering someone's brain, damaging the tiny vessels surrounding the insula would be catastrophic. The insula is "kind of a treacherous region actually to sample," says Damisah, among the first to forge ahead.

The procedure has two steps. First, while a patient is awake, Damisah robotically places electrodes deep inside the brain. Partly she's waiting for a seizure to occur naturally so she can watch how it moves through the patient's brain. But being able to access this area of the brain while a person is alive and awake is so novel in itself that the electrodes also help her learn more about what the elusive insula actually does.

Damisah says many of her patients' seizures make them feel crazy—their bodies suddenly get hot, they experience untethered distressing emotions, or in LaRock's case a low moan turned

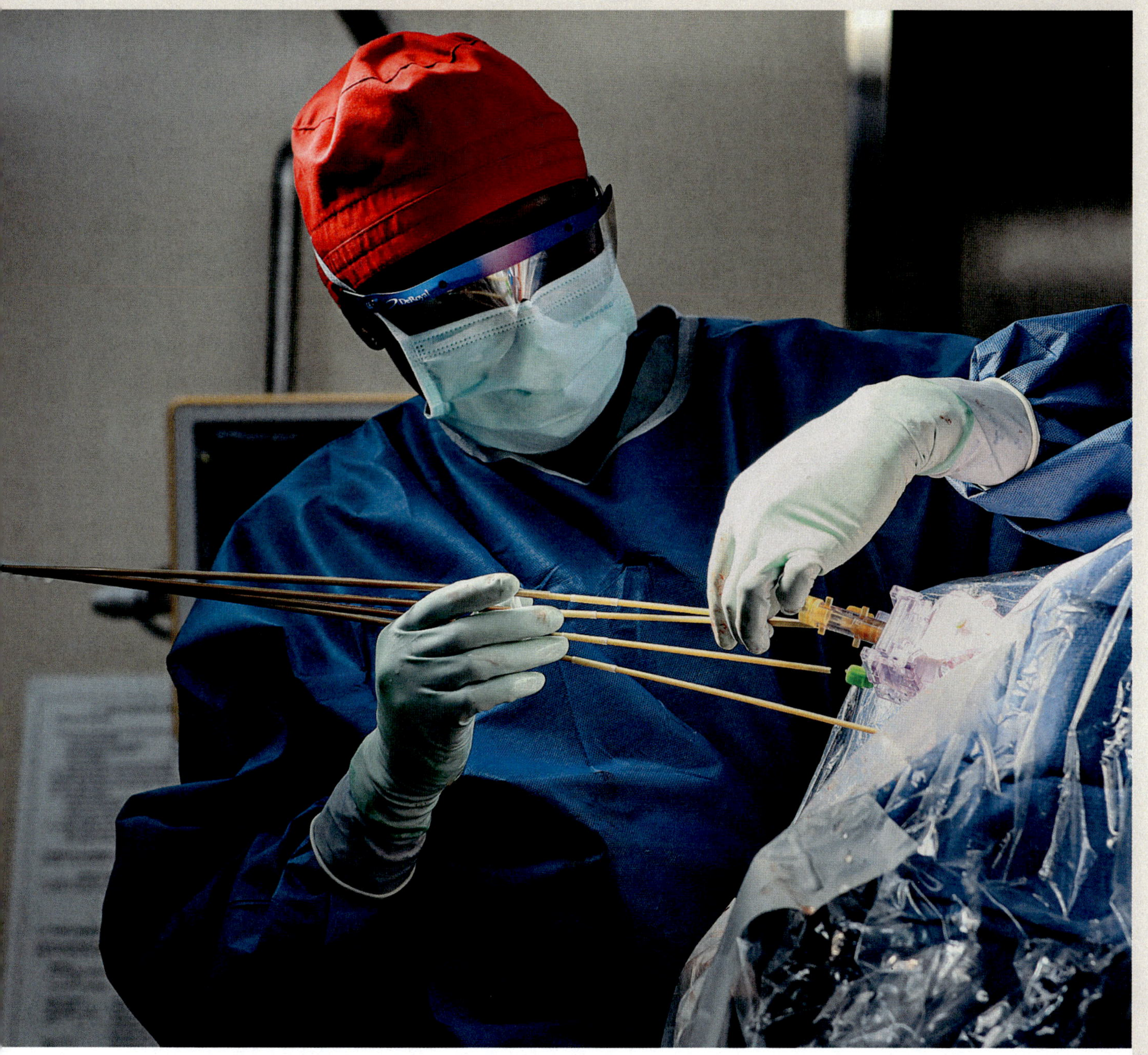

Neurosurgeon Eyiyemisi Damisah (above and left) is pioneering techniques to extract parts of the insula, a deep brain structure implicated in consciousness and severe cases of epilepsy. Here she preps a patient for surgery.

into a full-blown scream as she got older. "The insula, the way I look at it, is like a compact brain itself," she says. "All the functions you have in the big cortex, you actually have a lot of those in the insula." So, unusual seizure symptoms may actually be a sign of epilepsy originating inside the insula. After the electrode diagnosis and placement are complete, the patient will return for the second surgery, during which they're unconscious, and Damisah removes a small sample of the insula as a seizure-busting method.

She believes this tricky little structure to be the origin of many kinds of seizures that spread throughout the brain and remain unresponsive to other surgeries and medications. So far, post-surgery, LaRock has been seizure free.

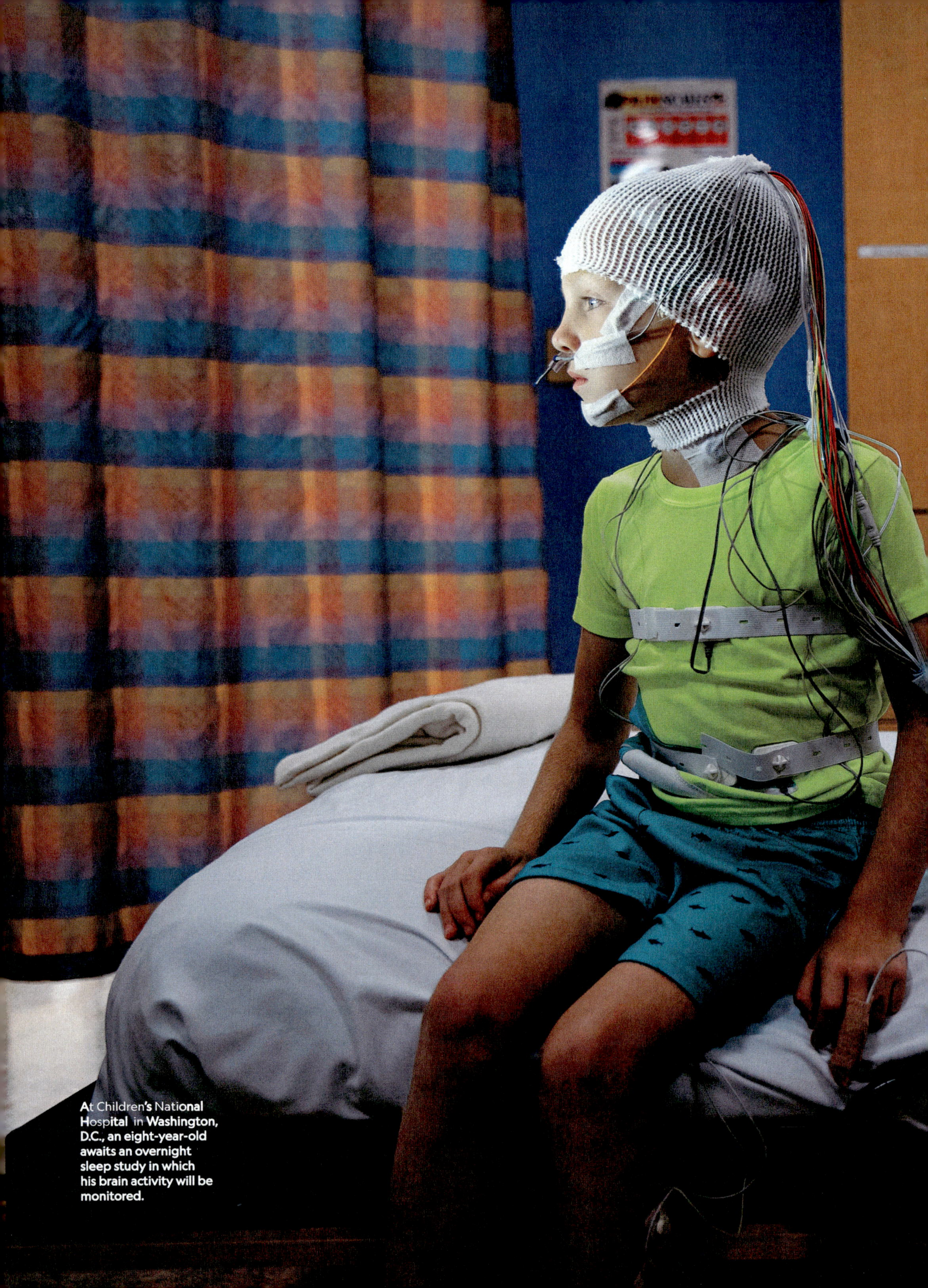

At Children's National Hospital in Washington, D.C., an eight-year-old awaits an overnight sleep study in which his brain activity will be monitored.

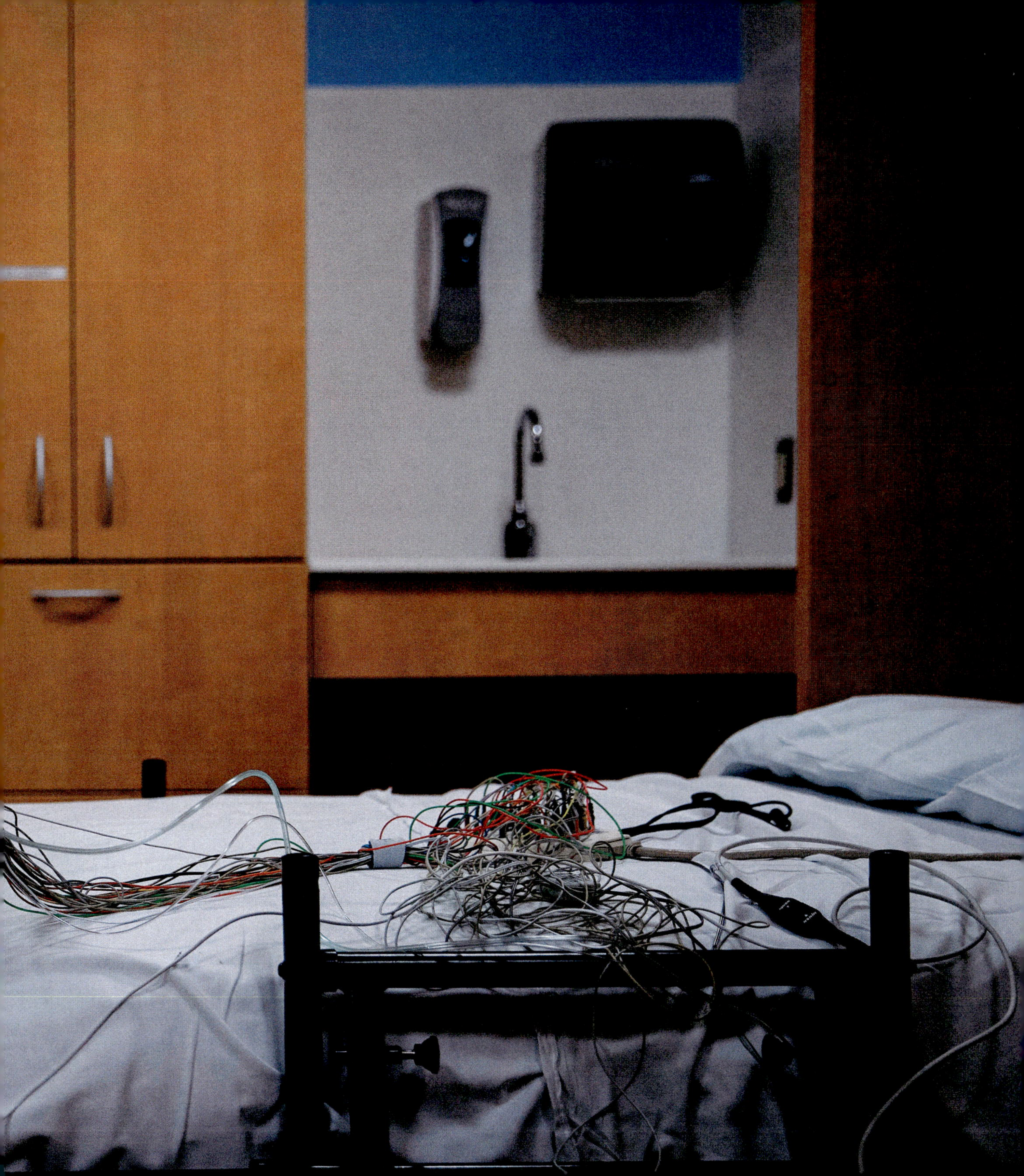

NO SEAT OF CONSCIOUSNESS

IN 2016, A simple finding in the brainstem took the popular press by storm—the seat of consciousness had been found! Five years later, Athena Demertzi, a cognitive and clinical neuroscientist, laughs about this. While based at the Université de Liège, in Belgium, Demertzi was recruited to work on a study with a group of researchers based mainly at Harvard University. She was looking to identify specific brain lesions that cause coma, a temporary state of unconsciousness that's devastating, and not well understood.

After carefully imaging the brains of coma patients—who are difficult to find and fragile to work with—she and the team compared these brainstems with those of conscious patients who

Athena Demertzi inspects brain scans of patients with a diverse array of consciousness disorders. Some scans show brain trauma, while others show lack of oxygen to the brain.

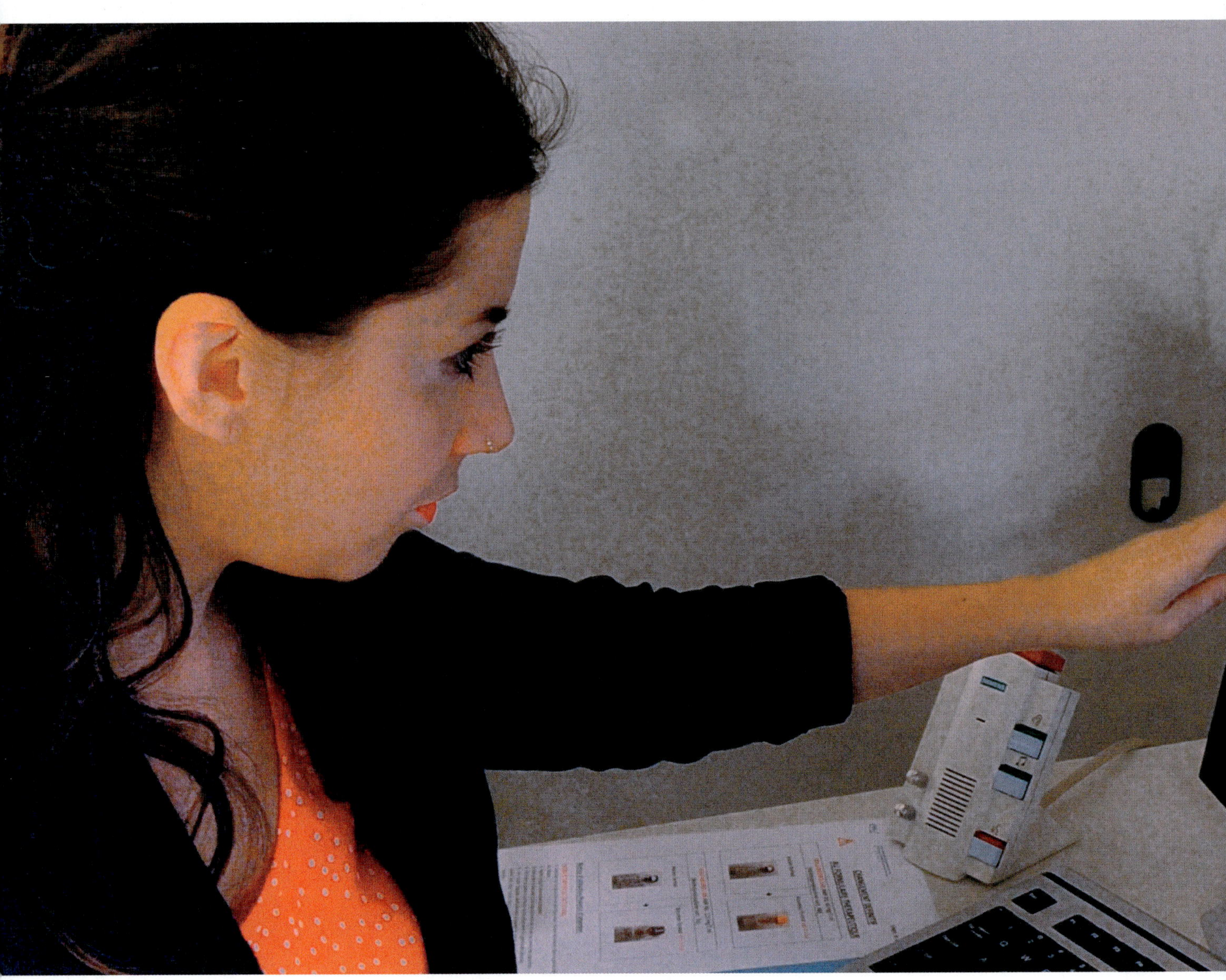

also had brainstem lesions. In coma patients, the team found that a tiny lesion in a piece of the brainstem, a critical structure that forms the bridge between body and brain, seemed to be bringing down a whole network: The pontine tegmentum appeared disconnected from the anterior insula and the anterior cingulate cortex, a network that *maintains* consciousness—maintains being the operative word.

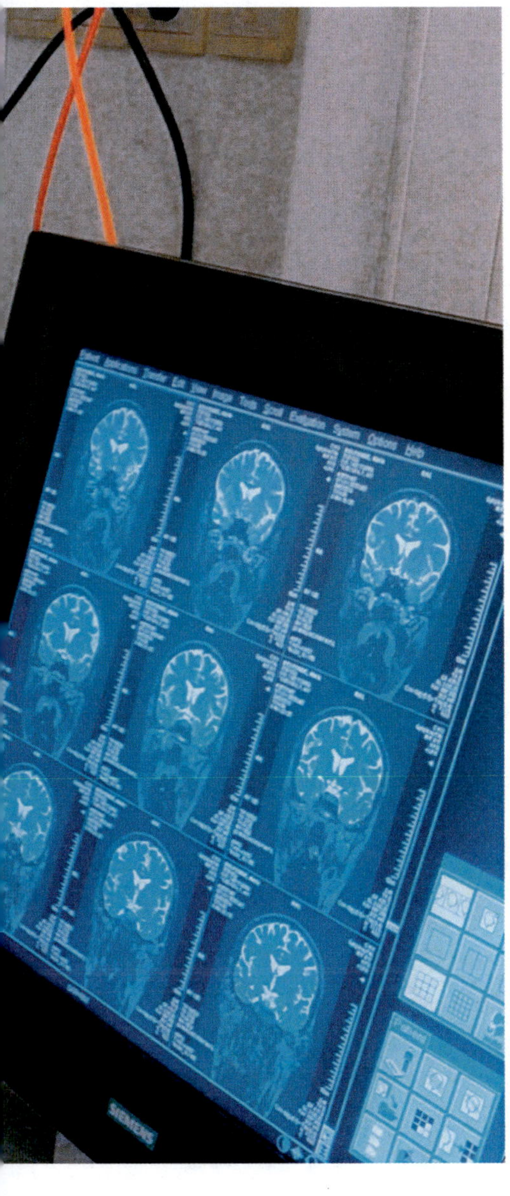

"It just put the seat [of consciousness] into conversations," says Demertzi, but she cautions that you can't draw any major conclusions about the finding from such a correlative approach with a small number of patients. Although a localized source of consciousness has certainly not been found, having even this level of insight into how comatose states come on—and could potentially be reversed—is pretty rare.

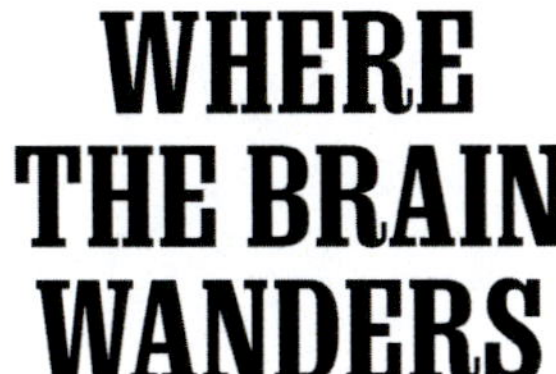

WHERE THE BRAIN WANDERS

DEMERTZI IS ONE of the scientists who thinks that consciousness is the product of the brain reacting to the environment, not a sense that arises unprompted from within itself. The question of where consciousness comes from is too hypothetical. Instead, she turns her attention back to those so-called easy problems, and to correcting an imbalance in brain imaging studies.

The way she sees it, so many investigations into brain imaging are related to tasks, or functional experiences: What network in the brain activates when you see a face? How about when you eat or smell something? And when you're in pain? These studies are important for understanding how big cognitive processes take shape, such as memory, learning, attention, or emotion. This research has also been crucial in reframing the brain as an organ

While we doze, the brain's immune cells, called microglia, come in to clean up the mess we made during the day.

not made of distinct functional areas, but of shifting networks that alternately kick into action or get pushed to the back burner, depending on what's happening in our environment.

What the brain does on its own time is far more mysterious. Imaging studies that attempt to understand the brain during a neutral resting state show that even when we externally appear to be doing nothing, the brain is busy. "Even during resting state . . . your mind still wanders," Demertzi says. "It goes here, there, everywhere—into the future and into the past. This is supported somehow. It has neural correlates, this resting state."

BUT THE BRAIN cannot always be this on. We know this because we go to sleep every day partly to let the brain refresh. While we doze, the brain's immune cells, called microglia, come in to clean up the mess we made during the day. What Demertzi is working on now is understanding whether there are times when consciousness shuts off in a healthy person's brain, but not as a function of coma or sleep. Yes, the mind sometimes wanders when there's no specific task going on, but sometimes it also seems to just . . . stop. Then something snaps you back into the here and now, and you have no idea where you've been. Colloquially called mind-blanking, no one knows what this looks like neurobiologically. "This, for me, is very, very intriguing, because it would mean that you don't have to be unconscious only when your arousal is low," Demertzi says. "You can really be unconscious while your eyes are open and you move around."

A recent EEG study found that during wakeful mind-blanking, the brain exhibits the kind of low-wave activity that normally happens during sleep. Demertzi wants to see if this holds up in fMRI studies. Her long-term goal is to apply her findings to developing preclinical predictors of who might develop neurodegenerative diseases that also seem to alter someone's conscious experience of the world, such as Alzheimer's.

LIKE DEMERTZI, MOST researchers who are deep in the neuronal weeds think the hard problem of consciousness—why we have self-awareness in the first place—is fundamentally unanswerable, which is incredible to think about. "I don't know why we have it," says Demertzi. "I think, personally, it's an evolutionary accident that we are both cursed and blessed to have."

There's some final frontier that our strong, complex brains can't reason through. They compose music, bring us to outer space, create groundbreaking vaccines in the middle of a pandemic; they make memories and create flavor. But at the deepest level, it seems a brain can't follow its own consciousness to the end of the trail.

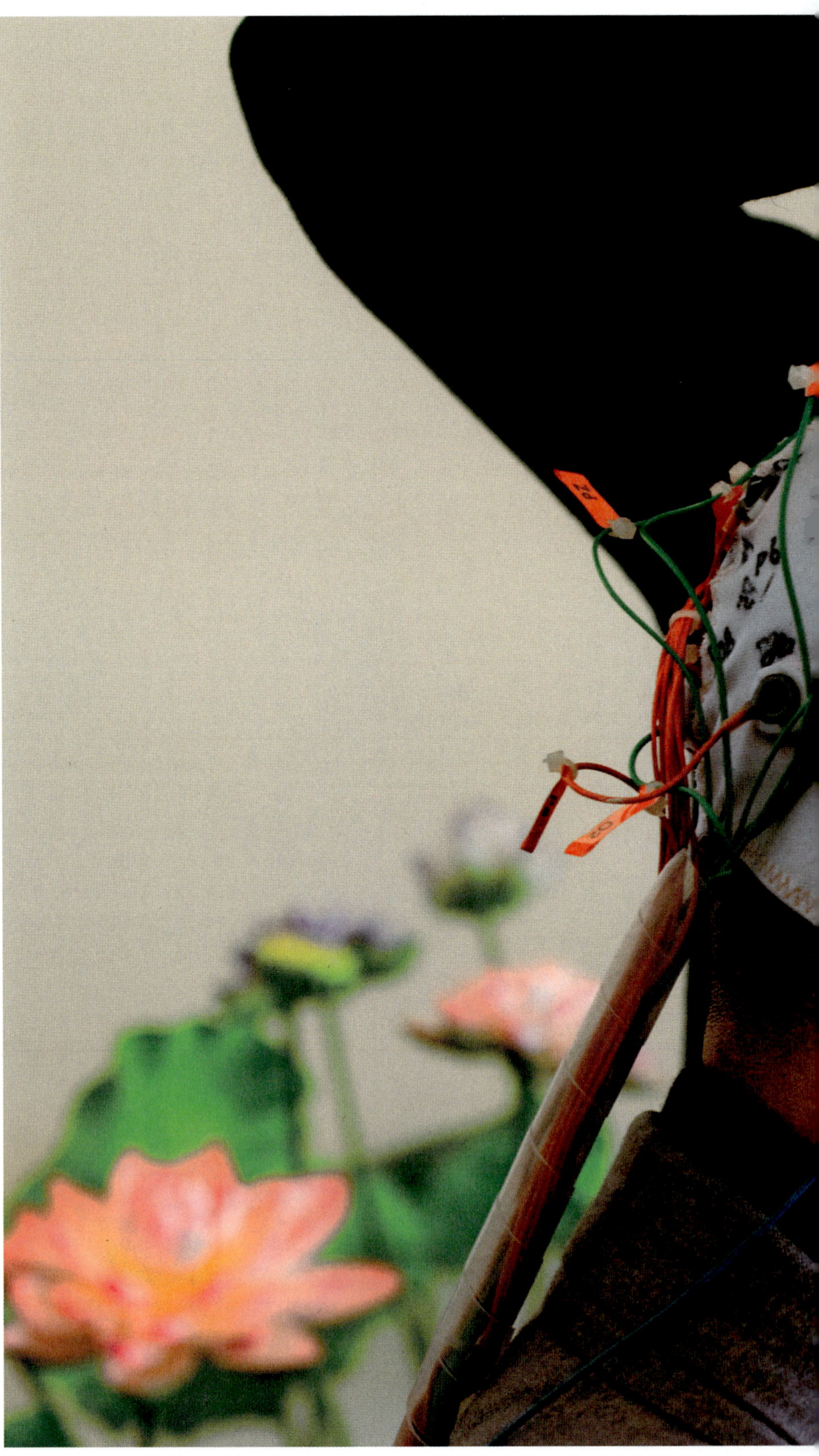

Electrodes measure the brain activity of a meditating Buddhist monk in Dengfeng, Zhengzhou, Henan Province, China.

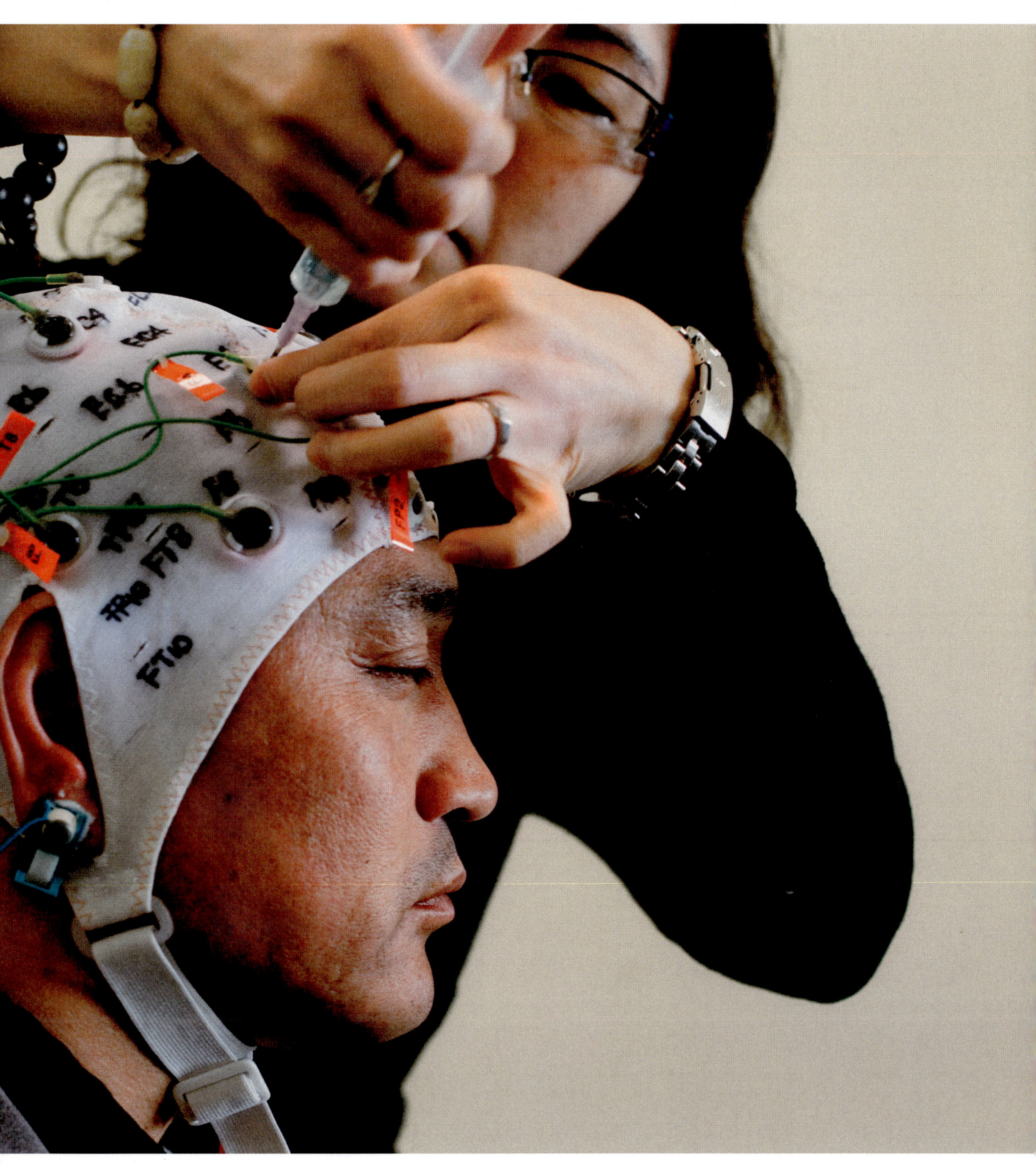
FT8
FT10

THE BRAIN

Julia Sklar

PRODUCED BY
NATIONAL GEOGRAPHIC PARTNERS, LLC
1145 17th Street NW
Washington, DC 20036-4688 USA

ISSN 2160-7141

Published by Meredith Operations Corporation
225 Liberty Street • New York, NY 10281

Printed in the USA

Special thanks to Mary Norris, Jill Foley, Becky Lang, Marshall Kiker, Mesa Schumacher, Justin Cook, and Alyssa Schukar. Additional thanks to Christine Ann Denny, Regan Fry, Chris White, Joe DeGutis, Mary Bichner, Akiko Okifuji, and Eyiyemisi Damisah.

Julia Sklar is an award-winning science journalist. She reports on health, food innovation, and medical technology as they intersect with people's lives. Her reporting has appeared in *National Geographic*, the *Boston Globe*, and many other publications. She lives in Boston. Find her on Twitter @ByJuliaSklar

ILLUSTRATIONS CREDITS

Cover, Alfred Pasieka/Science Source; 0–1, Lucas Foglia/National Geographic Image Collection; 2–3, Steve Raymer/National Geographic Image Collection; 4, Sherbrooke Connectivity Imaging Lab/Science Source; 9, Heritage Images/Getty Images; 10, Alyssa Schukar for National Geographic; 11, Alyssa Schukar for National Geographic; 12 (UP LE), Martin Schoeller/National Geographic Image Collection; 12 (UP CTR), Martin Schoeller/National Geographic Image Collection; 12 (UP RT), Martin Schoeller/National Geographic Image Collection; 12 (CTR LE), Martin Schoeller/National Geographic Image Collection; 12 (CTR CTR), Martin Schoeller/National Geographic Image Collection; 12 (CTR RT), Martin Schoeller/National Geographic Image Collection; 12 (LO LE), Martin Schoeller/National Geographic Image Collection; 12 (LO CTR), Martin Schoeller/National Geographic Image Collection; 12 (LO RT), Martin Schoeller/National Geographic Image Collection; 13 (UP LE), Martin Schoeller/National Geographic Image Collection; 13 (UP CTR), Martin Schoeller/National Geographic Image Collection; 13 (UP RT), Martin Schoeller/National Geographic Image Collection; 13 (LO LE), Martin Schoeller/National Geographic Image Collection; 13 (LO LE), Martin Schoeller/National Geographic Image Collection; 14, Justin Cook for National Geographic; 15, Sabine Scheckel/Getty Images; 16, Regan Fry; 17, Polina Shuvaeva/Getty Images; 18, Rebecca Hale/National Geographic Image Collection; 19, National Geographic/Ben Spaner; 20, Justin Cook for National Geographic; 21, Mary Bichner; 22–23, Jonathan Beckley; 24 (UP), Paul Matzner/Alamy Stock Photo; 24 (LO), Mary Bichner; 25, Daniel Mullen and Lucy Cordes Engelman; 26, Horst Tappe/Hulton Archive/Getty Images; 27, Roger Harris/Science Source; 28 (UP), Edward M. Hubbard,A. Cyrus Arman,Vilayanur S. Ramachandran; 28 (LO), USC Stevens Neuroimaging and Informatics Institute for the Human Connectome Project; 29, Jose Luis Pelaez Inc/Getty Images; 31, Andrew Stewart/robertharding.com; 32, Brian Finke c/o Everybody Somebody, Inc/National Geographic Image Collection; 33, Brian Finke/National Geographic Image Collection; 35, Brian Finke c/o Everybody Somebody, Inc/National Geographic Image Collection; 36–37, Brian Finke c/o Everybody Somebody, Inc/National Geographic Image Collection; 38–39, Alejandro Pagni/Getty Images; 40, Steve Gschmeissner/Science Source; 41, Heinz/Getty Images; 42, Igor Madjinca/Stocksy; 43, Steve Gschmeissner/Science Source; 44, Claus Frantzen/Courtesy of Qian Janice Wang; 45, Mateusz Tarkowski/Courtesy of Qian Janice Wang; 46 (LE), Rebecca Hale/National Geographic Image Collection; 46 (RT), Rebecca Hale/National Geographic Image Collection; 47, Brian Finke/National Geographic Image Collection; 48, Prostock-studio/Shutterstock; 49, David Zendle; 51, MagicTorch, Ltd.; 52, Bruna Bortolato/National Geographic Image Collection; 53, F. Astier/MetroDoloris/Science Source; 54–55, David Guttenfelder/National Geographic Image Collection; 56, James King-Holmes/Science Source; 57, Erika Larsen/National Geographic Image Collection; 58, Shannon Fagan/Getty Images; 59, M. I. Walker/Science Source; 60–61, Robert Clark/National Geographic Image Collection; 62, Mary Turner/The New York Times/Redux Pictures; 63, Kamila Lozinska; 64, Ann McKee, MD, VA Boston Healthcare/BU CTE Center; 65, Kalman Zabarsky for Boston University Photography; 66, Stan Grossfeld/The Boston Globe/Getty Images; 67, RealPeopleGroup/iStock/Getty Images; 70, Shiho Fukada/The New York Times/Redux Pictures; 71, Alexey Kuzma/Stocksy; 72, Stan Grossfeld/The Boston Globe/Getty Images; 73, Stan Grossfeld/The Boston Globe/Getty Images; 75, Sam Hundley/National Geographic Image Collection; 76–77, Eric Kayne; 78, Greg Dunn and Brian Edwards; 79, Eric Kayne; 82, akg-images; 83, Program for Translational Brain Mapping, Department of Neurosurgery, University of Rochester Medical Center; 84, agsandrew/Shutterstock; 85, James King-Holmes/Henry Luckhoo/Science Source; 86, Mikaël Theimer; 87, James King-Holmes/Science Source; 88, Jenny Chen; 89, Jenny Chen; 90–91, Magnus Wennman/National Geographic Image Collection; 92–93, Dr Raimondo Federico/Courtesy of Athena Demertzi; 94–95, Fritz Hoffman/National Geographic Image Collection; 97, Science History Images/Alamy Stock Photo.

Opposite: Santiago Ramon y Cajal's turn of the 20th-century drawings of microscopic neurons paved the way for modern neuroscience.

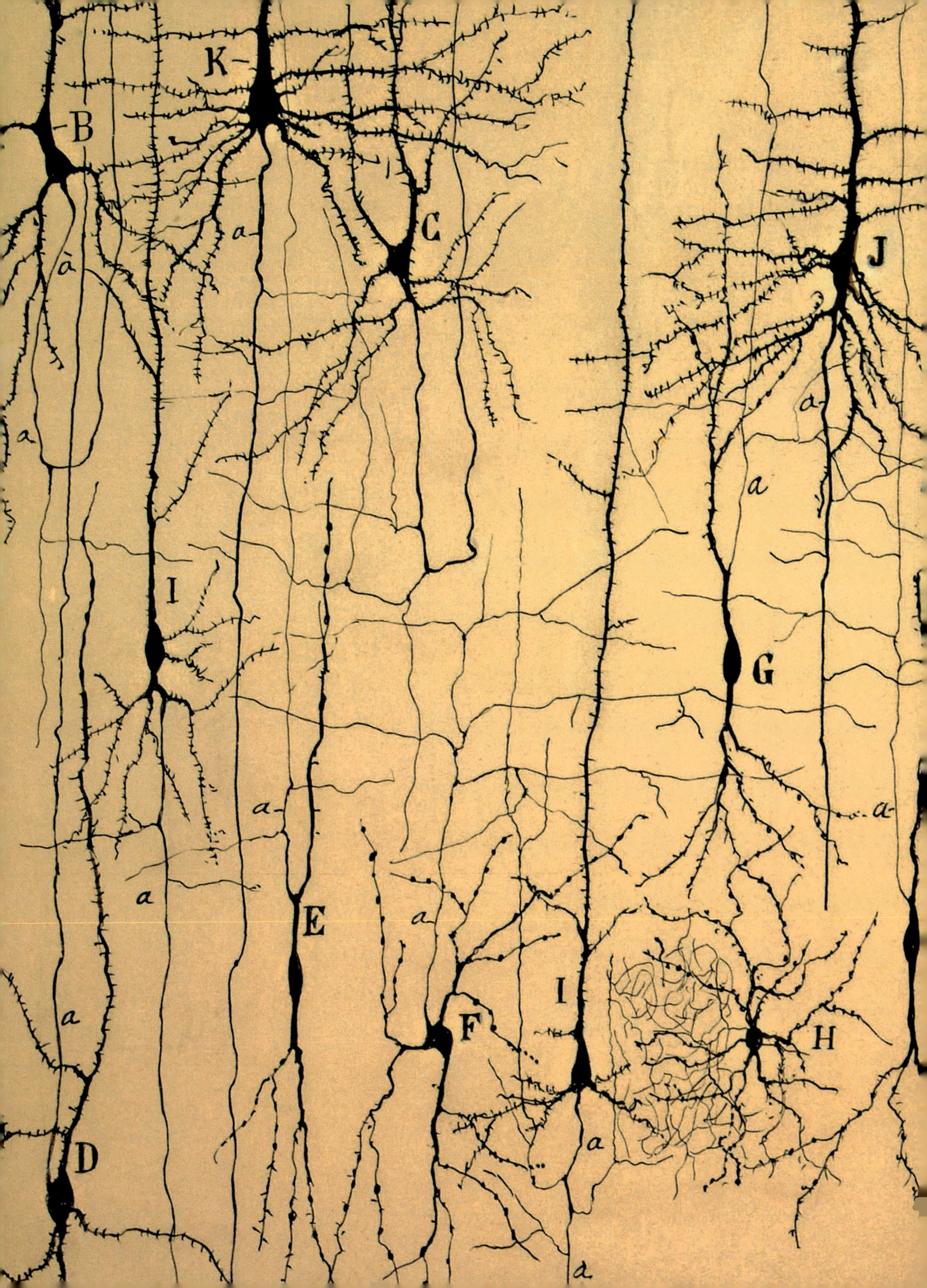
K
B
C
J
a
I
G
E
F
I
H
D

Made in the USA
Las Vegas, NV
08 June 2022

49971627R00059